Cannabis Strains for the Modern Professional: A Guide to Boosting Productivity and Wellness

Dr. Marlo Richardson

Table Of Contents

Chapter 1: Understanding
Cannabis and its Effects on
Productivity and Wellness   5

Chapter 2: The Benefits of
Cannabis for Professional
Productivity and Wellness   12

Chapter 3: Navigating the
World of Cannabis Strains   19

Chapter 4: Selecting the Right
Cannabis Strains for
Professional Success   28

Chapter 5: Incorporating Cannabis into Your Professional Lifestyle 37

Chapter 6: Legal and Ethical Considerations for Professionals 46

Chapter 7: Resources and Recommendations for Cannabis Strain Selection 54

Conclusion: Embracing Cannabis as a Tool for Professional Success and Wellness 63

Looking Ahead 70

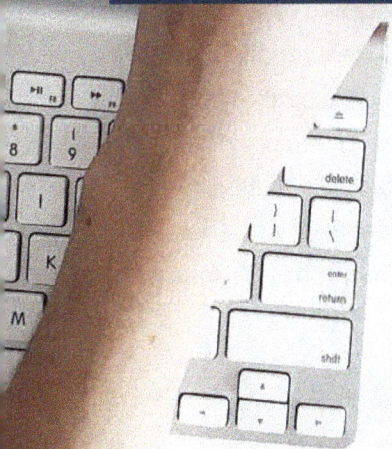

In the grand tapestry of human culture and natural wonders, cannabis holds a unique place. It is a plant that has been both revered and reviled, sought after for its medicinal properties and recreational allure, and yet, often misunderstood. As I set out to create this guide, my intention was not merely to catalog strains or to provide a handbook for cultivation. It was to weave together the story of cannabis, a narrative that spans thousands of years and touches every corner of the globe. This book is a testament to the plant's enduring legacy, its capacity to heal, and its power to bring joy and relaxation. My journey with cannabis began long before I decided to enter the industry or launch Just Mary Cannabis Brands. It started with curiosity, with questions that seemed to have as many answers as there were stars in the sky. What makes one strain different from another? How can the same plant elicit such a wide range of effects? And perhaps most intriguingly, how has something so natural become a point of contention in so many societies? These questions led me down a path of exploration, and what I discovered was a world rich with history, science, and an unwavering spirit of community. Cannabis, I learned, is more than just a plant. It is a reflection of humanity's relationship with nature, a tool for healing, and a source of creativity and relaxation. Its story is interwoven with our own, from ancient rituals to modern medicine, from prohibition to legalization. This book is my attempt to honor that story, to demystify the plant, and to provide a comprehensive guide that serves both novices and seasoned enthusiasts alike. The pages that follow are filled with the knowledge gathered from years of research, conversations with experts, and personal experience.

They offer a deep dive into the world of cannabis strains, exploring their origins, effects, and how they are cultivated. This guide also addresses the legal landscape, a crucial aspect for anyone looking to understand cannabis in today's world. It's designed to be informative, engaging, and above all, accessible, regardless of your familiarity with cannabis. But this book is also a call to action. It's an invitation to approach cannabis with an open mind and a critical eye. As the legal status of cannabis continues to evolve, so too must our understanding of it. We must challenge misconceptions, advocate for responsible use, and recognize the potential cannabis has to improve lives. Through education and conversation, we can shift the narrative around cannabis, focusing on its benefits and its place in a holistic approach to wellness. As you turn these pages, I invite you to join me on this journey. Whether you're looking to learn about the different strains, curious about cultivation, or seeking to understand the broader cultural and legal implications of cannabis, there's something in this guide for you.

It is my sincere hope that this book not only answers your questions but also inspires new ones, encouraging you to explore the ever-expanding world of cannabis. Marlo Richardson To continue from here, the next steps would involve diving into the detailed content of the guide, starting with the fundamental aspects of cannabis and moving through strain profiles, cultivation tips, and legal considerations.

In my previous life, the world of cannabis was one I observed from the periphery, often through the lens of law enforcement and regulatory frameworks. As a former police lieutenant and someone appointed by the Governor of California to oversee aspects of public safety, my interactions with cannabis and those who used it were, by necessity, dictated by the letter of the law. It was a perspective grounded in duty and often, in the misconceptions and stigmas that have historically surrounded cannabis use. My journey from that point to where I stand today—deeply immersed in the cannabis industry, advocating for its benefits and pioneering Just Mary Cannabis Brands—has been transformative, not just for me but for my understanding of this complex and often misunderstood plant. This transformation began with a personal story, one that unfolded in the quiet and privacy of my family home. It was my mother who unknowingly guided me onto this new path. Watching her struggle with chronic pain was heart-wrenching.

The options available through traditional medicine were often accompanied by a host of undesirable side effects, leaving her caught between the agony of her condition and the toll of her treatments. It was a no-win situation that I felt powerless to change, until we discovered the potential of cannabis, not as a recreational substance, but as a medicinal aid. The turning point came with a simple cannabis-infused salve. Skeptical but desperate for relief, we were astounded by the results. Here was a natural, non-intrusive remedy that managed her pain without the side effects that had made her other medications intolerable. This experience was a revelation. It challenged everything I thought I knew about cannabis, prompting me to delve deeper into its medicinal properties, its history, and the science behind its effects. Armed with this new knowledge and driven by a desire to share it, I transitioned from my role in law enforcement to become an advocate and entrepreneur in the cannabis industry. This book is a culmination of that journey. It's more than just a guide to cannabis strains or a manual on cultivation; it's a testament to the plant's versatility and its potential to improve lives. It's an invitation to view cannabis through a new lens, informed by both science and personal experience.

In these pages, I share not only the knowledge I've accumulated about cannabis strains, their effects, and how they're grown but also the broader context of cannabis as medicine and a cultural phenomenon.

From the personal to the professional, my journey reflects a broader shift in perception towards cannabis, one that recognizes its value beyond the recreational, as a source of relief and wellness. But this book is also a call to action. It's an encouragement to approach cannabis with an open mind and a critical eye, to educate oneself about its benefits and potential risks. It's a plea for empathy for those who, like my mother, turn to cannabis as a last resort in their search for relief. And it's a challenge to the stigma and misconceptions that still surround cannabis use, even as legal barriers begin to fall.

As you embark on this journey with me, I hope you find not only useful information but also a new perspective on cannabis. Whether you're a seasoned user, a curious newcomer, or someone skeptical of cannabis's place in medicine and society, there's something in this guide for you. Together, we can navigate the complex world of cannabis, armed with knowledge, compassion, and an open heart.

01

Chapter 1: Understanding Cannabis and its Effects on Productivity and Wellness

The History and Cultural Significance of Cannabis

Cannabis, also known as marijuana, has a rich history that dates back thousands of years. This subchapter aims to explore the historical and cultural significance of cannabis, shedding light on its origins and the impact it has had on various societies throughout time. Understanding the roots of this plant can help us appreciate its potential benefits and how it has become an integral part of modern society.

Ancient civilizations, such as the Chinese, Egyptians, and Indians, were among the first to recognize the medicinal properties of cannabis. In China, it was used for its pain-relieving and anti-inflammatory effects, while in ancient Egypt, it was valued for its psychoactive properties and was even used during religious ceremonies. The Indian subcontinent gave birth to the concept of "ganja," a term that refers to the consumption of cannabis for spiritual enlightenment and relaxation.

Moving forward in history, cannabis made its way to the Americas through European explorers and colonizers. It became an essential crop for early settlers due to its versatility as a source of fiber, food, and medicine. However, as time progressed, cannabis faced increasing scrutiny and legal restrictions, leading to its classification as a controlled substance in the 20th century.

Despite the legal challenges, cannabis has maintained its cultural
significance, particularly within countercultures and subcultures. It
became associated with artistic expression, rebellion, and the
pursuit of freedom. From the beatniks of the 1950s to the hippies
of the 1960s and beyond, cannabis played a central role in shaping
the cultural landscape of these eras.

Today, as we enter a new age of cannabis legalization and
acceptance, it is important to recognize the potential benefits of
this plant beyond recreational use. Cannabis has shown promise in
managing various medical conditions, such as chronic pain,
epilepsy, and anxiety. Moreover, it has gained traction as a wellness
tool, with professionals turning to specific strains to boost
productivity, focus, and overall well-being.

By understanding the history and cultural significance of cannabis, we can appreciate how it has evolved and adapt it to the needs of the modern professional. This guide aims to provide insights into different cannabis strains and their potential benefits, helping professional men and women aged 30-75 navigate the ever-expanding world of cannabis products and make informed decisions on how to incorporate it into their lives for increased productivity and wellness.

Cannabis Basics: THC, CBD, and Other Cannabinoids

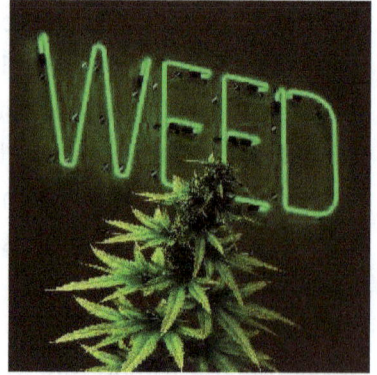

Understanding the basics of cannabis is essential for anyone looking to explore its potential benefits for productivity and wellness. In this subchapter, we will delve into the key components of cannabis - THC, CBD, and other cannabinoids - to help professional men and women aged 30-75 navigate the world of cannabis strains.

Cannabis Strains for the Modern Professional: A Guide to Boosting Productivity and Wellness

THC, or tetrahydrocannabinol, is one of the most well-known cannabinoids found in cannabis. It is responsible for the psychoactive effects commonly associated with marijuana. While THC can induce a feeling of euphoria and relaxation, it may also impair cognitive function and cause anxiety in some individuals.

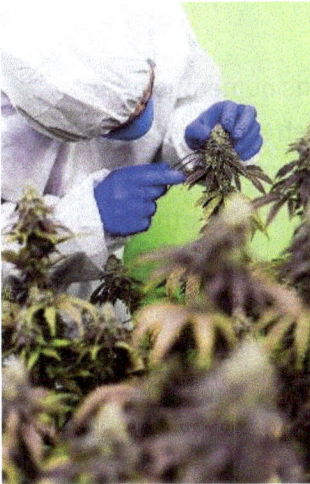

For professionals seeking to enhance productivity, strains with lower THC levels may be more suitable, allowing them to experience the potential benefits of cannabis without compromising their focus or mental clarity.

On the other hand, CBD, or cannabidiol, is gaining popularity for its potential therapeutic properties. Unlike THC, CBD does not produce a high but has been linked to various wellness benefits. It is known to have anti-inflammatory, analgesic, and anxiolytic properties, making it an appealing option for individuals seeking relief from stress, chronic pain, or anxiety. CBD-rich strains with minimal THC content are often preferred by professionals who want to experience the potential therapeutic effects of cannabis without the psychoactive side effects.

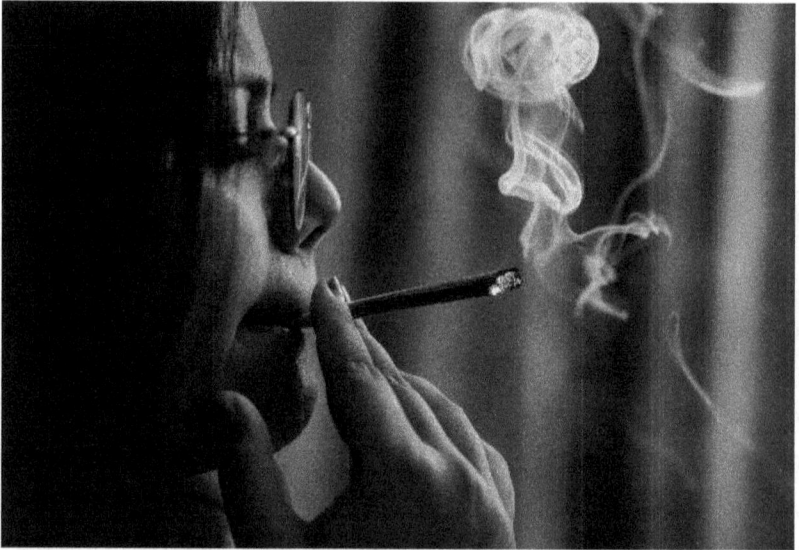

Apart from THC and CBD, cannabis contains numerous other cannabinoids that contribute to its overall effects. These cannabinoids include CBG (cannabigerol), CBC (cannabichromene), and CBN (cannabinol), among others. Each cannabinoid has unique properties and potential benefits, which is why understanding their presence and concentrations in different strains is crucial for professionals seeking specific outcomes.

By exploring the diverse cannabinoid profiles of cannabis strains, professionals can tailor their cannabis experience to suit their individual needs. Whether you are looking for relaxation after a long day, relief from chronic pain, or a boost in creativity and focus, there is likely a strain with the right cannabinoid composition to support your goals.

In the following chapters, we will provide a comprehensive cannabis strain guidebook, detailing various strains, their cannabinoid profiles, and recommended uses for professional men and women seeking to maximize productivity and wellness in their daily lives. Stay tuned to discover the perfect cannabis strain to enhance your professional journey.

The Science of Cannabis: How it Interacts with the Body

In recent years, there has been a surge of interest in the potential health benefits of cannabis. From relieving chronic pain to reducing anxiety, this versatile plant has captured the attention of professionals seeking alternative wellness solutions. But how does cannabis actually work within the body? Understanding the science behind its interactions is crucial for harnessing its full potential.

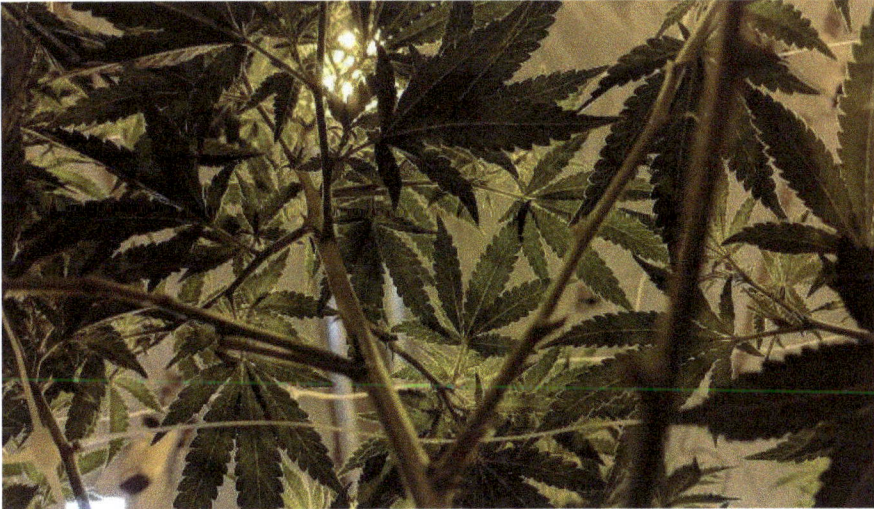

Cannabis Strains for the Modern Professional: A Guide to Boosting Productivity and Wellness

At the heart of cannabis' effects lies a complex network of receptors called the endocannabinoid system (ECS). Discovered in the late 1980s, the ECS plays a pivotal role in maintaining homeostasis in the body. It consists of receptors, endocannabinoids produced by the body, and enzymes that regulate their activity.

When cannabis is consumed, its active compounds, known as cannabinoids, interact with the ECS. The most well-known cannabinoids are tetrahydrocannabinol (THC) and cannabidiol (CBD). THC is responsible for the psychoactive effects commonly associated with cannabis, while CBD is non-intoxicating and may offer various therapeutic benefits.

When THC enters the body, it binds to the ECS receptors, primarily found in the brain and immune system. This interaction triggers a cascade of effects, leading to the well-known sensations of euphoria and relaxation. CBD, on the other hand, does not directly bind to these receptors but modulates their activity, potentially providing relief from pain, inflammation, and anxiety.

The specific effects of cannabis can vary greatly depending on the strain. Different strains have varying levels of THC and CBD, as well as other beneficial compounds like terpenes. These compounds work synergistically in what is known as the entourage effect, enhancing the overall therapeutic potential of the plant.

For professional men and women aged 30-75, understanding the science behind cannabis is essential for making informed decisions about which strains to incorporate into their wellness routine. A comprehensive cannabis strain guide book can provide valuable insights into the various strains available and their potential benefits. By choosing strains tailored to their specific needs, professionals can boost productivity, enhance relaxation, and promote overall wellness.

It is important to note that cannabis affects individuals differently, and finding the right strain and dosage may require some experimentation. Consulting with a healthcare professional experienced in cannabis therapeutics can provide personalized guidance and ensure safe and effective cannabis use.

As the modern professional seeks natural alternatives to enhance their productivity and wellness, understanding the science of cannabis and its interactions with the body is a crucial step towards harnessing its full potential. With the right knowledge and guidance, professionals can confidently navigate the world of cannabis strains and unlock the numerous benefits this remarkable plant has to offer.

Debunking Myths and Misconceptions about Cannabis

In recent years, the perception of cannabis has undergone a significant transformation. As more states and countries legalize its use for medical and recreational purposes, it is crucial to separate fact from fiction when it comes to this versatile plant. In this subchapter, we aim to debunk common myths and misconceptions surrounding cannabis, providing professional men and women aged 30-75 with accurate information to make informed decisions about its use.

Myth #1: Cannabis is a gateway drug
One of the most persistent myths about cannabis is that it serves as a gateway drug, leading to the use of more dangerous substances. However, numerous scientific studies have disproven this notion. Research shows that the majority of cannabis users do not progress to harder drugs and that individual predisposition, environment, and social factors play a more significant role in substance abuse.

Myth #2: Cannabis makes you lazy and unmotivated
Contrary to popular belief, cannabis can actually enhance productivity and motivation when used appropriately. Different strains and dosages can provide energizing effects that boost focus, creativity, and overall mood. Cannabis can be integrated into a professional's routine to enhance their well-being, helping them maintain a healthy work-life balance.

Myth #3: Cannabis causes memory loss and cognitive impairment
While it is true that cannabis can affect short-term memory and cognitive abilities temporarily, the notion that it causes long-term damage has been largely debunked. Studies indicate that any cognitive impairments are typically reversible and diminish once cannabis use is discontinued. Moreover, some strains actually have neuroprotective properties, potentially benefiting brain health.

Myth #4: All cannabis strains have the same effects
The vast array of cannabis strains available can be overwhelming for newcomers. It is essential to dispel the misconception that all strains have identical effects. Cannabis contains various compounds, such as cannabinoids and terpenes, which contribute to different effects. Understanding the nuances of different strains and how they can be tailored to specific needs is crucial for achieving desired outcomes.

By debunking these myths and misconceptions, we hope to empower professional men and women aged 30-75 to make informed decisions about cannabis use. It is important to approach this plant with an open mind, recognizing its potential benefits and understanding the role it can play in enhancing productivity and wellness. With the right knowledge, individuals can navigate the world of cannabis strains confidently, unlocking its potential to support their professional and personal lives.

02

Chapter 2: The Benefits of Cannabis for Professional Productivity and Wellness

The Role of Cannabis in Reducing Stress and Anxiety

In today's fast-paced and demanding world, stress and anxiety have become common issues faced by professionals across various industries. The pressures of work, family, and personal life can take a toll on our mental well-being, affecting our productivity and overall quality of life. However, there is a natural solution that has gained significant recognition in recent years – cannabis.

This subchapter explores the role of cannabis in reducing stress and anxiety, providing valuable insights for professional men and women aged 30 to 75 who are seeking a natural and effective way to manage their daily stressors.

Cannabis, when used responsibly and in moderation, has shown promise in alleviating symptoms of stress and anxiety. The plant contains various chemical compounds, including cannabinoids, such as THC and CBD, that interact with our body's endocannabinoid system. This system plays a crucial role in regulating stress responses and mood.

By targeting specific receptors in the brain, cannabis can help to calm the mind, promote relaxation, and reduce anxiety levels. It has been observed that certain strains of cannabis can have more pronounced effects in these areas. Our guidebook provides a comprehensive cannabis strain guide, allowing you to choose the most suitable strains for your specific needs and preferences.

Moreover, cannabis can enhance the body's ability to cope with stress by promoting quality sleep. Sleep deprivation is a common consequence of stress and anxiety, exacerbating their effects. Cannabis strains with sedative properties can help improve sleep quality, allowing professionals to wake up refreshed and ready to face the day.

It is important to note that cannabis affects individuals differently, and finding the right strain and dosage is crucial. The guidebook includes detailed information on different strains, their effects, and recommended dosages, helping professionals make informed decisions about incorporating cannabis into their wellness routines.

As a natural alternative to pharmaceuticals, cannabis offers a holistic approach to reducing stress and anxiety. By harnessing its potential, professionals can experience a greater sense of well-being, improved productivity, and a better work-life balance. So, whether you are an executive, entrepreneur, or creative professional, this subchapter will empower you to navigate the world of cannabis strains, enabling you to discover how they can become a valuable tool in your pursuit of productivity and wellness. Embrace the power of cannabis and take control of your stress and anxiety today!

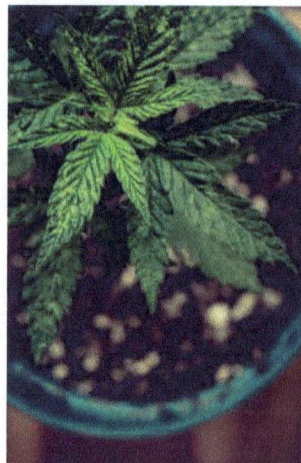

Enhancing Focus and Concentration with Cannabis

Cannabis Strains for the Modern Professional: A Guide to Boosting Productivity and Wellness

In today's fast-paced and demanding professional world, maintaining focus and concentration is crucial for success. With the growing acceptance and legalization of cannabis, many professionals are turning to this natural plant to enhance their productivity and overall wellness.

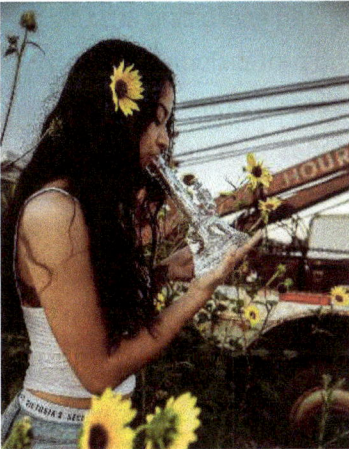

In this subchapter, we will explore how specific cannabis strains can help professional men and women aged 30-75 improve their focus and concentration, ultimately boosting their productivity and overall success in the workplace.

Strains for Enhanced Focus: Not all cannabis strains are created equal when it comes to improving focus and concentration. Some strains are known to induce relaxation and promote sleepiness, while others have energizing and stimulating effects. For professionals looking to enhance their focus, it is important to choose strains that can provide mental clarity without causing sedation.

Cannabis Strains for the Modern Professional: A Guide to Boosting Productivity and Wellness

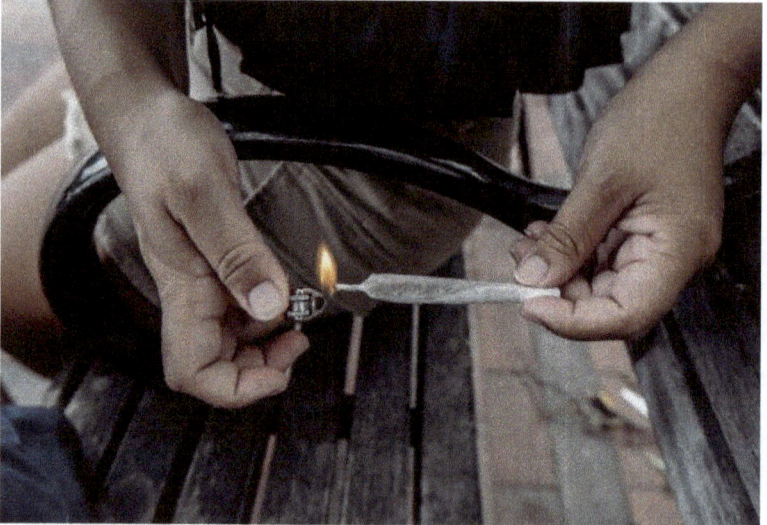

1. Durban Poison: Known for its uplifting and energizing effects, Durban Poison is a popular choice among professionals seeking improved focus and concentration. This sativa-dominant strain promotes mental clarity, creativity, and focus without the unwanted side effects of drowsiness or mental fog.

2. Green Crack: Despite its name, Green Crack is a strain that offers a burst of mental energy and focus, making it ideal for professionals who need to stay alert and productive throughout the day. This sativa-dominant strain is known to boost motivation, creativity, and mental clarity.

3. Jack Herer: Named after the renowned cannabis activist, Jack Herer is a strain that provides a clear-headed and focused high. This sativa-dominant hybrid offers an uplifting and energizing effect, enabling professionals to stay sharp and focused on their tasks.

Using Cannabis Responsibly:

While cannabis can offer significant benefits for enhancing focus and concentration, it is essential to use it responsibly. Professionals should always be mindful of their dosage and consumption method to avoid impairing their cognitive abilities or becoming excessively sedated. It is advisable to start with low doses and gradually increase as needed to find the optimal level of focus and concentration enhancement.

C

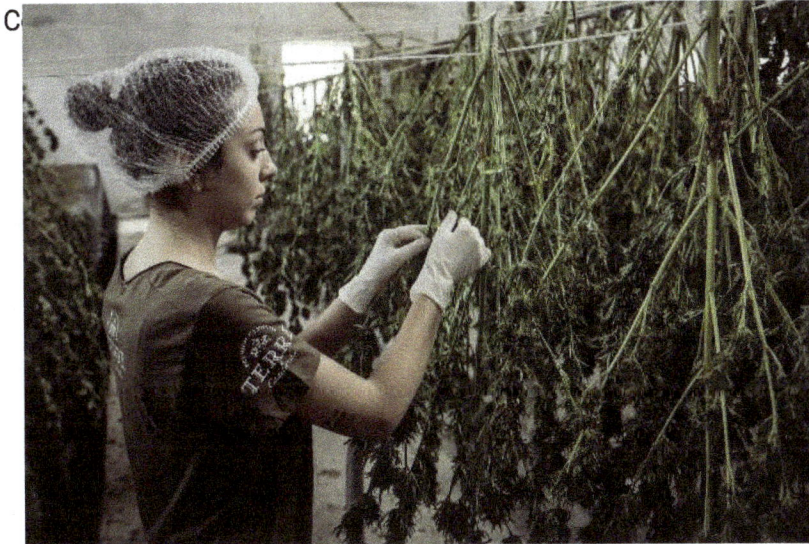

In the fast-paced world of professionals, maintaining focus and
concentration is paramount. Cannabis strains like Durban Poison,
Green Crack, and Jack Herer can provide professionals aged 30-75
with the mental clarity and energy needed to excel in their careers.
However, it is essential to use cannabis responsibly, starting with
low doses and finding the right strain that suits individual needs.
By incorporating cannabis into their wellness routine, professional
men and women can unlock their full potential and achieve greater
productivity and success in their professional lives.

Boosting Creativity and Problem-Solving Abilities

In today's fast-paced and highly competitive professional world,
creativity and problem-solving abilities are essential skills for
success. As a professional, you are constantly faced with
challenges that require innovative thinking and unique solutions.
To stay ahead of the game, you need to tap into your creative
potential and enhance your problem-solving abilities. Surprisingly,
one tool that can help you achieve this is cannabis.

In this subchapter, we will explore how different cannabis strains
can boost your creativity and problem-solving skills, providing you
with a unique edge in your professional endeavors. Whether you're
a seasoned cannabis user or new to the world of cannabis, this
guide will help you navigate the vast array of strains available and
find the perfect match for your needs.

Cannabis has long been known to enhance creativity by stimulating the brain's creative centers. It can help you think outside the box, make connections between seemingly unrelated ideas, and inspire innovative solutions. Different strains have varying levels of THC and CBD, which produce different effects on the brain. We will delve into the science behind these effects and provide practical advice on selecting the right strain for your creative pursuits.

Moreover, cannabis can also improve problem-solving abilities by promoting focus and reducing stress and anxiety. By calming the mind and allowing you to fully immerse yourself in the task at hand, cannabis can enhance your ability to tackle complex problems and find effective solutions. We will explore strains that are particularly beneficial for problem-solving, providing you with a comprehensive understanding of how cannabis can optimize your cognitive functioning.

Additionally, we will discuss responsible cannabis use in a professional setting, ensuring that you maintain productivity and professionalism while harnessing the benefits of cannabis. With guidelines on dosage, timing, and consumption methods, you will be able to integrate cannabis into your routine effectively, maximizing its potential without compromising your work performance.

Whether you're an artist seeking inspiration, an entrepreneur looking for innovative business ideas, or a corporate professional aiming to enhance your problem-solving skills, this subchapter will equip you with the knowledge and tools to leverage the power of cannabis and boost your creativity and problem-solving abilities. Remember, cannabis is a tool that should be used responsibly and with awareness. By exploring the world of cannabis strains and understanding their effects on your cognitive abilities, you can unlock your full creative potential and become a more effective problem solver in your professional life.

Cannabis for Physical Wellness and Pain Management

In recent years, the perception of cannabis has shifted dramatically. Once considered a recreational drug, it is now recognized for its potential to enhance physical wellness and manage pain. This subchapter will explore the benefits of cannabis strains specifically tailored for the modern professional, providing a comprehensive guide to boosting productivity and overall well-being.

Understanding Physical Wellness:
Physical wellness is crucial for professionals of all ages. It encompasses various aspects, including fitness, nutrition, and mental health. Cannabis can play a significant role in promoting physical wellness by alleviating pain, reducing inflammation, and aiding in relaxation.

Pain Management with Cannabis:
Chronic pain affects millions of individuals, making it difficult to focus, perform daily tasks, and maintain a high quality of life. Cannabis strains rich in CBD (cannabidiol) have shown promising results in managing pain, without the psychoactive effects commonly associated with THC (tetrahydrocannabinol). This subchapter will provide detailed information on specific strains that are effective for various types of pain, such as migraines, arthritis, and muscle soreness.

Reducing Inflammation:
Inflammation is a common underlying factor in many health conditions, including autoimmune diseases, chronic pain, and even mental health disorders. Cannabis strains with anti-inflammatory properties can help reduce inflammation, providing relief and improving overall physical wellness. This section will explore the best strains for inflammation, highlighting their unique properties and potential benefits.

Enhancing Relaxation and Sleep:
In today's fast-paced world, professionals often struggle with
stress, anxiety, and sleep disorders. Cannabis strains with relaxing
qualities can offer a natural alternative to pharmaceutical
medications. By calming the mind and promoting deep, restful
sleep, these strains can significantly improve physical wellness.
The subchapter will include strain recommendations for relaxation
and sleep enhancement, along with important considerations and
potential side effects.

Conclusion:
Cannabis strains tailored for physical wellness and pain
management have the potential to revolutionize the lives of
modern professionals. By incorporating these strains into their
daily routines, professionals can experience enhanced productivity,
reduced pain, and overall improved well-being. This subchapter
serves as a comprehensive guide, providing valuable information
on strains, their properties, and how they can be utilized by
professional men and women aged 30-75 to achieve optimal
physical wellness.

03

Chapter 3: Navigating the World of Cannabis Strains

Indica vs. Sativa: Understanding the Differences

When it comes to cannabis strains, the two most common types you'll encounter are Indica and Sativa. These terms refer to the different species of the Cannabis plant and can have distinct effects on the body and mind. As a professional looking to incorporate cannabis into your life, it's vital to understand the differences between Indica and Sativa to make informed choices about which strains are best suited for your needs.

Indica strains are known for their relaxing and sedative properties. They typically have higher levels of CBD (cannabidiol) and lower levels of THC (tetrahydrocannabinol), the compound responsible for the psychoactive effects of cannabis. Indica strains are often associated with feelings of calmness, pain relief, and can be beneficial for those dealing with anxiety, insomnia, or muscle tension. These strains are great for unwinding after a long day or promoting restful sleep.

On the other hand, Sativa strains are known for their uplifting and energizing effects. They tend to have higher levels of THC and lower levels of CBD. Sativa strains often provide a cerebral and creative high, boosting focus, motivation, and productivity.

They are great for daytime use, helping you stay alert and engaged without feeling weighed down. Sativa strains can also enhance mood and alleviate symptoms of depression or fatigue, making them an excellent choice for those seeking a productivity boost or a creative spark.

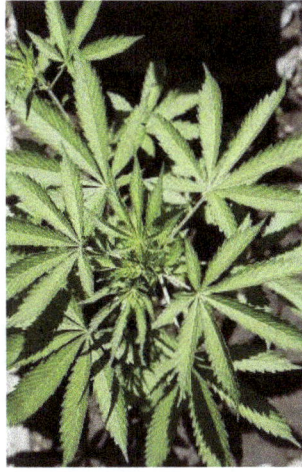

It's important to note that many cannabis strains available today are hybrids, combining the characteristics of both Indica and Sativa strains. These hybrid strains offer a wide range of effects and can be tailored to suit individual preferences and needs. Whether you're looking for relaxation, pain relief, enhanced focus, or a balanced experience, there is likely a hybrid strain that fits the bill.

Cannabis Strains for the Modern Professional: A Guide to Boosting Productivity and Wellness

When selecting a cannabis strain, it's crucial to consider your desired outcomes and the specific effects you're seeking. Experimenting with different strains and keeping track of how they affect you personally can help you find the perfect strain to boost your productivity and overall wellness.

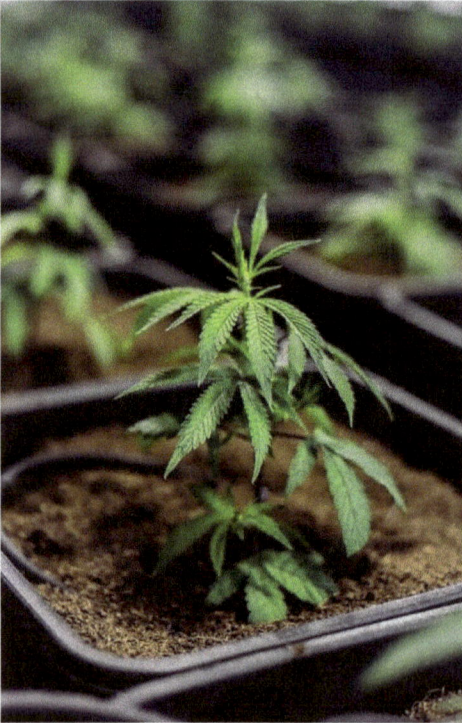

In conclusion, understanding the differences between Indica and Sativa strains is essential for professionals looking to incorporate cannabis into their lives. While Indica strains offer relaxation and pain relief, Sativa strains provide an uplifting and energizing experience. Hybrid strains, combining the best of both worlds, offer a range of effects to suit individual needs.

By exploring and experimenting with different strains, professionals can find the perfect cannabis companion to enhance their productivity and overall well-being.

Hybrid Strains: Finding the Perfect Balance

In the world of cannabis, hybrid strains have gained immense popularity due to their ability to offer the best of both worlds. Whether you are a professional man or woman, aged 30-75, looking to enhance your productivity and overall wellness, understanding hybrid strains is essential. This subchapter aims to provide you with valuable insights on how to find the perfect balance with hybrid strains, guiding you through the vast array of options available in the market.

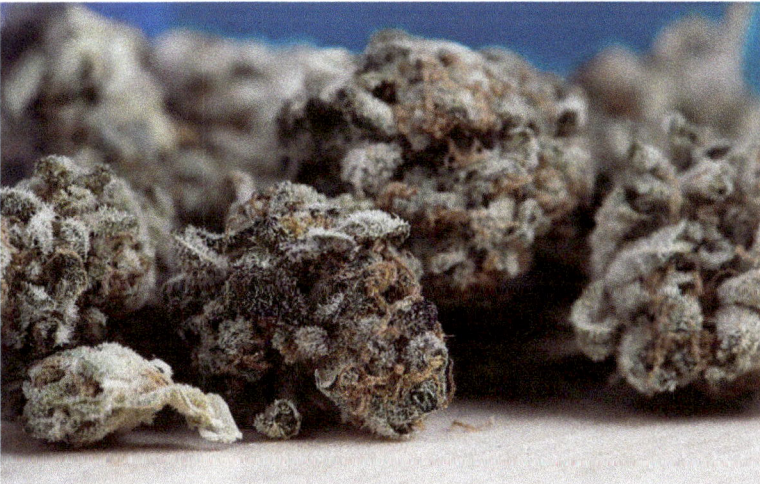

Cannabis Strains for the Modern Professional: A Guide to Boosting Productivity and Wellness

Hybrid strains are the result of crossing two or more cannabis varieties, combining the desirable characteristics of both. This unique blending allows for a more personalized experience, catering to your specific needs and preferences. While sativa strains are known for their energizing effects, and indicas for their relaxing properties, hybrids offer the ideal middle ground. They can provide a gentle uplift, enhancing focus, creativity, and productivity, while simultaneously offering a sense of calm and relaxation.

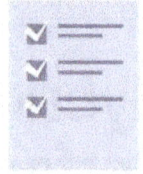

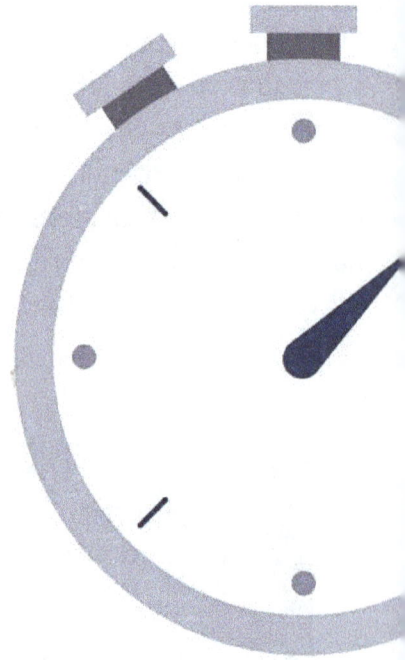

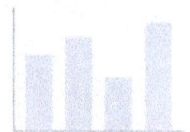

Cannabis Strains for the Modern Professional: A Guide to Boosting Productivity and Wellness

When selecting a hybrid strain, it is crucial to consider the ratio of sativa to indica genetics. This ratio plays a significant role in determining the overall effects. For instance, a strain with a higher sativa percentage will provide more energizing and uplifting effects, perfect for daytime use when you need a mental boost.

On the other hand, strains with a higher indica ratio offer a more calming and sedating experience, ideal for unwinding after a long day or promoting restful sleep.

To further personalize your experience, hybrid strains also come with a diverse range of terpene profiles. Terpenes are aromatic compounds found in cannabis, responsible for its unique flavors and scents. Each terpene profile offers distinct effects, such as increased focus, stress relief, or pain management. By exploring different terpene profiles, you can fine-tune your cannabis experience to suit your specific needs.

When incorporating hybrid strains into your wellness routine, it is vital to start low and go slow, especially if you are new to cannabis. Begin with a small dosage and gradually increase it until you find the perfect balance that suits your desired effects. Additionally, consulting with a knowledgeable budtender or a medical professional can provide valuable guidance and recommendations tailored to your individual needs.

In conclusion, hybrid strains offer a remarkable opportunity for professional men and women aged 30-75 to boost productivity and overall wellness. By understanding the different hybrid options available, considering the sativa to indica ratio, and exploring various terpene profiles, you can find the perfect balance that aligns with your lifestyle and goals. Remember to consume responsibly and enjoy the journey towards enhanced productivity and wellness with hybrid strains.

High-CBD Strains: Maximizing Wellness Benefits

In recent years, there has been a growing interest among professional men and women in using cannabis for its wellness benefits. As more and more states legalize the use of cannabis for medical and recreational purposes, individuals are discovering the myriad of ways in which this plant can enhance their overall well-being. One particular type of cannabis strain that has gained significant attention is high-CBD strains.

CBD, or cannabidiol, is a non-intoxicating compound found in cannabis that is known for its therapeutic properties. Unlike its counterpart THC, CBD does not produce the psychoactive effects commonly associated with consuming cannabis. Instead, it offers a range of potential wellness benefits such as reducing anxiety, alleviating pain and inflammation, improving sleep quality, and promoting a general sense of calm and relaxation.

For professional men and women, high-CBD strains can be particularly appealing as they provide the potential benefits of cannabis without impairing cognitive functions or inducing a feeling of being "stoned." This makes high-CBD strains an ideal choice for those seeking relief from stress, anxiety, or chronic pain, while still maintaining focus and productivity throughout the day.

When selecting a high-CBD strain, it is important to consider the specific wellness goals you wish to achieve. Different strains have varying CBD-to-THC ratios, and finding the right balance for your needs is essential. Some strains may contain equal amounts of CBD and THC, while others may have a higher CBD content and minimal THC. It's crucial to understand that the presence of THC can affect the overall experience, so it's recommended to start with strains that have lower THC levels if you are new to cannabis or have concerns about psychoactive effects.

In this subchapter, we will explore a comprehensive range of high-CBD strains tailored to meet the needs of professional men and women. We will delve into the specific wellness benefits associated with each strain and provide guidance on dosage, consumption methods, and potential side effects. Additionally, we will discuss the importance of lab-tested products and provide recommendations on reputable sources for obtaining high-quality high-CBD strains.

By incorporating high-CBD strains into your wellness routine, you can unlock the potential of cannabis to enhance your overall productivity, reduce stress, and promote a balanced and healthy lifestyle. Whether you are seeking relief from ailments or simply looking to optimize your well-being, this subchapter will serve as your ultimate guide to maximizing the wellness benefits of high-CBD strains.

Exploring Lesser-Known Cannabis Varieties

In the ever-expanding world of cannabis, there are countless strains to choose from. While popular varieties like OG Kush, Sour Diesel, and Blue Dream have gained widespread recognition, there is a whole universe of lesser-known cannabis varieties waiting to be explored. This subchapter aims to introduce you, professional men and women aged 30-75, to some of these hidden gems and shed light on their unique properties and potential benefits.

1. Lamb's Bread: Originating from Jamaica, Lamb's Bread is a sativa-dominant strain known for its uplifting and energizing effects. It can provide a boost of creativity and focus, making it an excellent choice for professionals looking to enhance their productivity and overall wellness.

2. Charlotte's Web: Named after a young girl named Charlotte who found relief from her seizures through this strain, Charlotte's Web is a CBD-dominant strain renowned for its therapeutic potential. It offers a gentle relaxation without the psychoactive effects of THC, making it suitable for those seeking relief from stress, anxiety, or chronic pain.

3. Durban Poison: This pure sativa strain hails from South Africa and is famous for its invigorating and clear-headed effects. Durban Poison can enhance focus, creativity, and productivity, making it an ideal choice for professionals who need a little extra motivation to tackle their day.

4. Harlequin: Another high CBD strain, Harlequin, offers a balanced ratio of CBD to THC. It provides a gentle relaxation while maintaining mental clarity, making it suitable for those looking to alleviate stress, anxiety, or inflammation without feeling overly sedated or impaired.

5. Green Crack: Despite its controversial name, Green Crack is a sativa-dominant strain that delivers a powerful burst of energy, focus, and mental clarity. It can be an excellent choice for professionals who need a pick-me-up during a long workday or for those seeking an alternative to caffeine.

By exploring these lesser-known cannabis varieties, you can expand your horizons and find strains that cater to your specific needs and preferences. Remember, it's always essential to start with low doses, experiment responsibly, and consult with a knowledgeable professional to ensure a safe and enjoyable experience.

In conclusion, this subchapter has introduced you to a selection of lesser-known cannabis varieties that can enhance productivity and wellness. As a professional, it's crucial to stay informed about the diverse range of strains available to optimize your cannabis experience and achieve the desired effects. Whether you seek relaxation, focus, or pain relief, these strains offer unique properties that may be just what you need to thrive in your personal and professional life.

04

Chapter 4: Selecting the Right Cannabis Strains for Professional Success

Identifying Personal Goals and Needs

In the fast-paced world of modern professionalism, it is crucial to take a step back and evaluate our personal goals and needs. As professional men and women aged 30-75, we often find ourselves caught up in the daily grind, neglecting our own well-being and happiness. This subchapter aims to guide you through the process of identifying your personal goals and needs, and how cannabis strains can play a role in enhancing your productivity and overall wellness.

Setting personal goals is essential for personal growth and fulfillment. Whether it's advancing in your career, maintaining a healthy work-life balance, improving your physical or mental health, or pursuing a passion project, identifying your goals allows you to focus your energy and efforts in the right direction. Within the pages of this book, you will find a comprehensive guide to various cannabis strains that can help support and amplify your journey towards achieving these personal goals.

Cannabis Strains for the Modern Professional: A Guide to Boosting Productivity and Wellness

Understanding your needs is equally important. Each one of us has unique needs when it comes to productivity and wellness. Some may require increased focus and concentration to excel in their professional endeavors, while others may seek stress relief or relaxation after a long day at work.

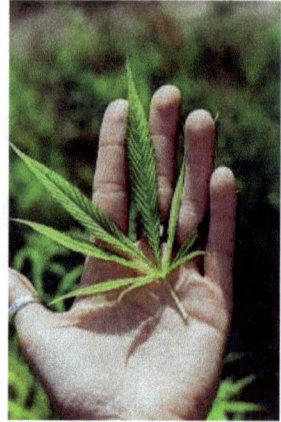

Through carefully curated strain recommendations and insights, this book will empower you to make informed choices that align with your individual needs.

By incorporating cannabis strains into your routine, you can unlock a world of possibilities for enhanced productivity and overall well-being. From strains that boost creativity and motivation to those that promote relaxation and stress relief, this subchapter will help you navigate through the vast array of options available.

Cannabis Strains for the Modern Professional: A Guide to Boosting Productivity and Wellness

You will gain a deeper understanding of the specific effects and benefits of different strains, enabling you to customize your cannabis experience to suit your personal goals and needs.

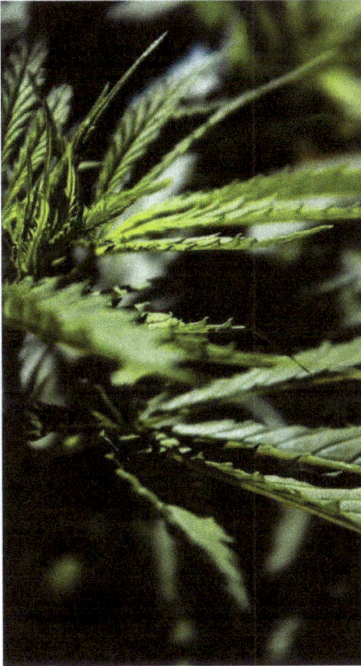

Remember, identifying personal goals and needs is an ongoing process. As you progress in your professional and personal life, your goals and needs may evolve, and so can your cannabis strain preferences. This book will serve as a valuable resource, providing you with the knowledge and tools to adapt and refine your approach to cannabis usage, ensuring a continued boost in productivity and wellness.

Embrace the power of cannabis strains for the modern professional, and embark on a journey towards achieving your personal goals, improving your overall well-being, and finding balance in your professional life.

Cannabis Strains for the Modern Professional: A Guide to Boosting Productivity and Wellness

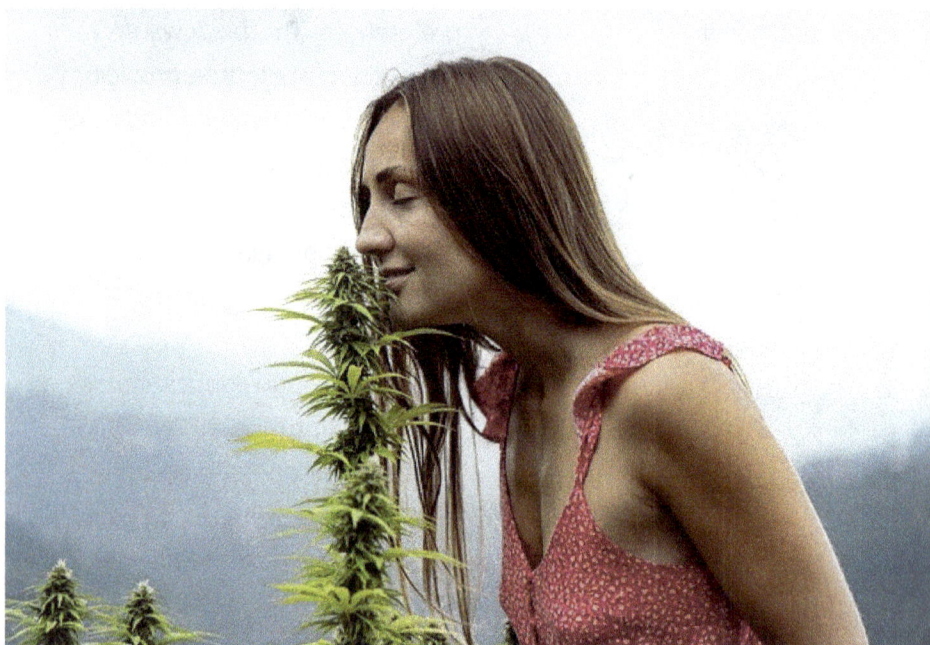

Matching Strains to Specific Professional Tasks and Situations

In today's fast-paced and demanding professional world, it is essential to find ways to enhance productivity and wellness. Cannabis, with its diverse range of strains and therapeutic properties, has emerged as a powerful tool for professionals looking to optimize their performance and well-being. This subchapter aims to guide professional men and women aged 30-75 through the process of matching cannabis strains to specific tasks and situations, ultimately boosting their productivity and overall quality of life.

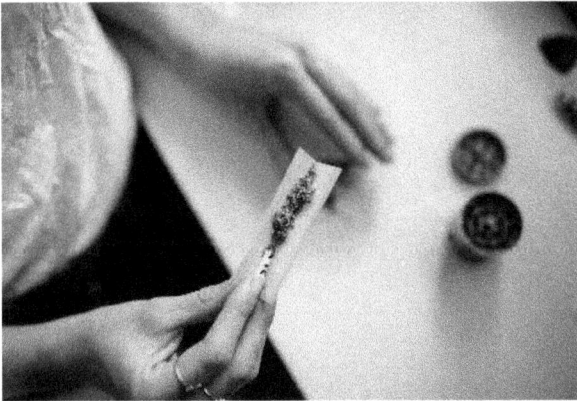

Cannabis Strains for the Modern Professional: A Guide to Boosting Productivity and Wellness

When it comes to selecting the right cannabis strain for a particular task or situation, it is crucial to consider individual preferences, desired effects, and the demands of the task at hand. For instance, if you are seeking enhanced focus and creativity for brainstorming sessions or creative work, strains with higher levels of THC and terpenes like Limonene or Pinene may be beneficial. These strains can stimulate creativity, uplift mood, and improve cognitive function.

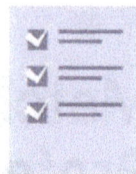

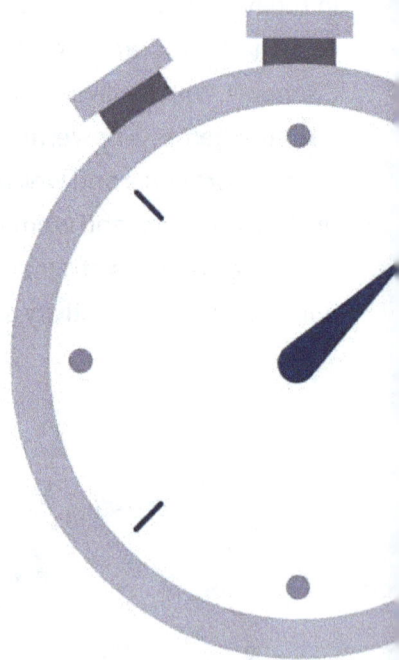

On the other hand, if you are dealing with high-stress situations, strains with higher CBD content and relaxing properties such as Myrcene or Linalool can help promote relaxation, reduce anxiety, and improve overall well-being. These strains can be particularly useful during important presentations, public speaking engagements, or high-pressure meetings.

Additionally, professionals who struggle with chronic pain, inflammation, or sleep disorders can benefit from strains rich in CBD and CBN. These cannabinoids have been shown to possess analgesic and sedative properties, helping individuals manage pain, reduce inflammation, and improve sleep quality. This, in turn, can lead to enhanced focus, improved mood, and increased productivity during work hours.

It is important to note that finding the right strain may require some experimentation and personalization. Every individual's body chemistry and tolerance levels are unique, so it is advisable to start with low doses and gradually increase as needed. Keeping a strain journal and noting down the effects of each strain can be instrumental in finding the perfect match for specific tasks and situations.

By understanding the different strains available and their effects, professional men and women can harness the power of cannabis to optimize their productivity, creativity, and overall well-being. This subchapter acts as a guide, helping professionals navigate the vast array of cannabis strains and empowering them to make informed choices that enhance their performance in the workplace and beyond.

Finding the Optimal Dosage for Productivity and Wellness

In the fast-paced world of modern professionals, maintaining productivity and wellness is crucial for success. With the increasing legalization and acceptance of cannabis, many individuals are turning to this plant as a tool to enhance their daily lives. However, understanding the optimal dosage of cannabis for productivity and wellness can be a challenging task. This subchapter aims to provide valuable insights and guidance to professional men and women aged 30-75, who are seeking to incorporate cannabis into their lives in a responsible and effective manner.

When it comes to cannabis, finding the right dosage is essential. Consuming too little may not yield the desired effects, while consuming too much can result in unwanted side effects, such as anxiety or lethargy. The key is to strike a balance that maximizes productivity and wellness without impairing cognitive function or hindering daily activities.

First and foremost, it is important to understand that everyone's body chemistry is unique. What works for one person may not work for another. Therefore, it is recommended to start with a low dosage and gradually increase it until you find the optimal level for your individual needs. Keeping a journal to track your experiences with different strains and dosages can be immensely helpful in determining what works best for you.

In the pursuit of productivity, certain cannabis strains are more suitable than others. Sativa-dominant strains, known for their energizing and uplifting effects, can provide a boost of focus, creativity, and motivation. However, it is crucial to find the right balance. Consuming too much of a stimulating strain may lead to restlessness or racing thoughts, ultimately hindering productivity. On the other hand, wellness encompasses both physical and mental wellbeing. Indica-dominant strains are renowned for their relaxation and pain-relieving properties. These strains can be beneficial for those seeking relief from stress, anxiety, or physical discomfort. However, it is important to be mindful of the sedating effects of indica strains, as excessive consumption can lead to drowsiness and reduced motivation.

Ultimately, finding the optimal dosage for productivity and wellness requires self-awareness, experimentation, and an understanding of the different cannabis strains available. It is crucial to approach cannabis consumption with a responsible mindset, respecting its potential effects and limitations.

This subchapter serves as a guide to help professional men and women navigate the world of cannabis strains, empowering them to make informed decisions that enhance their productivity and wellness. By finding the right dosage and strain, individuals can unlock the potential benefits of cannabis while maintaining their professional edge.

Considering Side Effects and Potential Risks

When it comes to exploring the world of cannabis strains for productivity and wellness, it is essential to be aware of the possible side effects and risks associated with their use. While cannabis has been proven to offer numerous benefits, it is important to approach its consumption with caution and understanding.

One of the most commonly known side effects of cannabis is the psychoactive effect, commonly referred to as a "high." This can vary depending on the strain and individual tolerance levels. While some professionals may find this effect enjoyable and even conducive to their work, it is crucial to be mindful of the potential impact it may have on productivity and cognitive abilities.

Another potential side effect to consider is the potential for addiction or dependency. While cannabis is not considered as addictive as other substances, it is possible for individuals to develop a psychological dependence on its use. It is important to monitor your consumption and ensure that it does not interfere with your daily life or responsibilities.

Additionally, cannabis may have various physical side effects that can range from mild to more severe. These can include dry mouth, red eyes, increased heart rate, dizziness, and impaired coordination. It is essential to be aware of these potential effects and adjust your usage accordingly to mitigate any negative impact on your professional life.

Furthermore, it is important to acknowledge that cannabis may interact with certain medications or medical conditions. If you have any preexisting health conditions or are taking medications, it is crucial to consult with a healthcare professional before incorporating cannabis into your wellness routine. They can provide guidance on potential interactions and help you make informed decisions.

Lastly, it is important to be mindful of the legal implications associated with cannabis use. Laws and regulations regarding cannabis can vary from region to region, so it is crucial to familiarize yourself with the applicable laws in your area. Understanding the legal landscape will help you make informed decisions and ensure you are compliant with local regulations.

In conclusion, while cannabis strains can offer numerous benefits for productivity and wellness, it is vital to consider the potential side effects and risks associated with their use. By being informed, cautious, and responsible, professional men and women can navigate the world of cannabis strains effectively, ensuring that they enhance their productivity and wellness without compromising their professional lives.

05

Chapter 5: Incorporating Cannabis Into Your Professional Lifestyle

Establishing Responsible Consumption Habits

In this subchapter, we will delve into the importance of establishing responsible consumption habits when it comes to cannabis use. While cannabis can offer numerous benefits for productivity and wellness, it is essential to approach its consumption with caution and mindfulness. This chapter aims to provide professional men and women, aged 30-75, with practical tips and guidelines to ensure responsible and safe cannabis use.

1. Understanding Your Goals and Intentions:
Before incorporating cannabis into your routine, it is crucial to identify your goals and intentions. Are you seeking enhanced focus, relaxation, or pain relief? By understanding your objectives, you can select the most appropriate cannabis strains that align with your needs.

2. Educate Yourself about Different Strains:
A responsible consumer is an informed consumer. Familiarize yourself with the various cannabis strains available and their specific effects. "Cannabis Strains for the Modern Professional" provides a comprehensive strain guide, detailing the characteristics and benefits of each strain, enabling you to make informed choices that suit your lifestyle and goals.

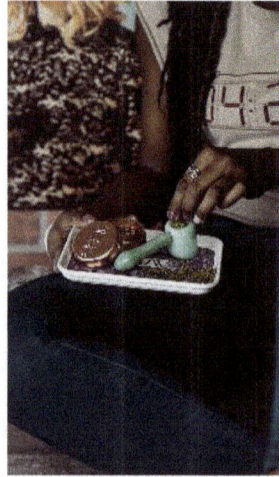

3. Start with Low Doses:
When trying a new cannabis strain, it is advisable to start with a low dose. This allows you to gauge your sensitivity to the strain and avoid any potential adverse effects. Gradually increase the dosage only if necessary, and always be mindful of your body's response.

4. Avoid Impairment during Work Hours:
As productive professionals, it is crucial to maintain focus and clarity during work hours. While cannabis can enhance creativity and productivity for many, it is essential to find the right balance. Avoid consuming cannabis immediately before or during work hours to prevent impairment that may hinder your performance.

5. Create a Routine and Set Boundaries:
Establishing a routine can help you maintain responsible cannabis use. Designate specific times for consumption, ensuring it does not interfere with your professional responsibilities or personal life. Set clear boundaries that enable you to enjoy the benefits of cannabis without encroaching on other aspects of your life.

6. Seek Professional Advice: If you are new to cannabis or have concerns about its potential interactions with medications or existing health conditions, consult a medical professional. They can provide personalized guidance and ensure you make informed choices that prioritize your health and well-being.

By establishing responsible consumption habits, you can maximize the benefits of cannabis while maintaining a productive and balanced professional life. Remember, moderation and mindfulness are key when incorporating cannabis into your routine. Embrace the guidance provided in this subchapter as you embark on a journey of enhanced productivity and wellness with cannabis strains tailored to the modern professional.

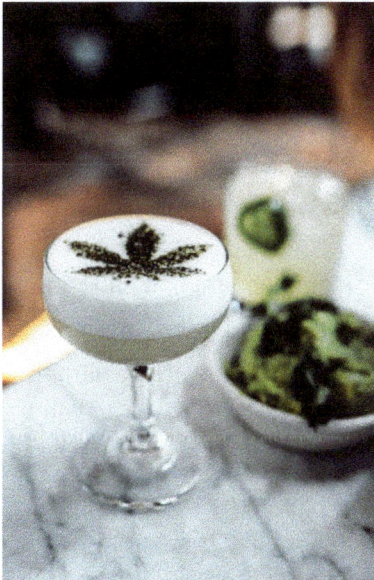

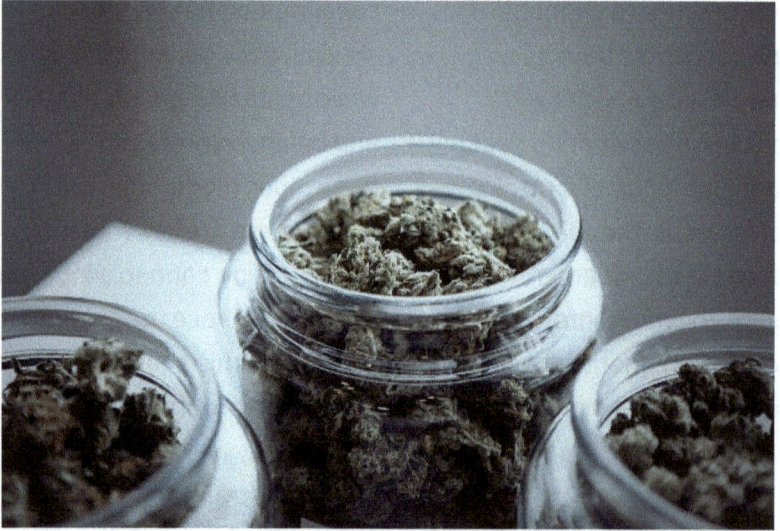

Tips for Using Cannabis At Work

In today's fast-paced professional world, finding ways to enhance productivity and maintain overall wellness is crucial. As cannabis becomes more widely accepted, many professionals are turning to this natural plant for its potential benefits. However, using cannabis at work requires careful consideration and responsible consumption. In this subchapter, we will explore some valuable tips to help professional men and women aged 30-75 enhance their work experience with cannabis while maintaining productivity and wellness.

Cannabis Strains for the Modern Professional: A Guide to Boosting Productivity and Wellness

1. Know your limits: It is essential to understand your tolerance and how cannabis affects you personally. Start with low doses and gradually increase until you find the right balance. This will prevent any unwanted side effects that could hinder your performance at work.

2. Choose the right strain: Cannabis strains vary in their effects, and some are better suited for work than others. Look for strains with uplifting and energizing properties, such as sativa-dominant hybrids. These strains can provide a boost of creativity, focus, and motivation without inducing sedation or impairing cognitive function.

3. Time your consumption: Plan your cannabis consumption strategically to align with your work demands. Consider using cannabis during breaks or after work hours to fully enjoy its effects without compromising your professional responsibilities. Remember, responsible consumption is key to maintaining productivity.

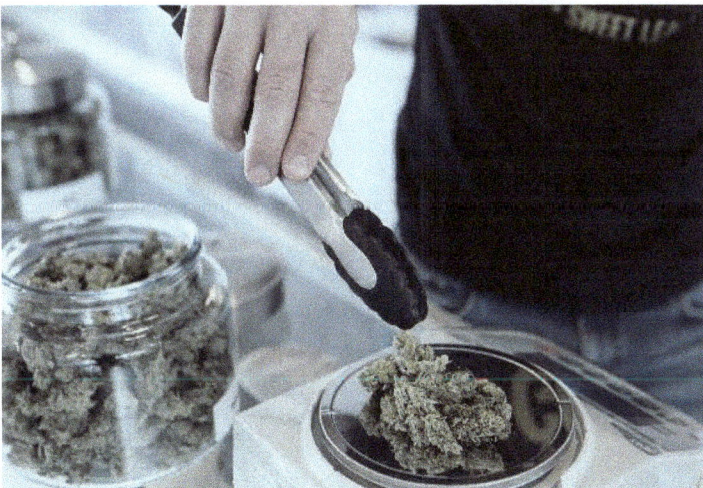

4. Be discreet: While cannabis is becoming more accepted, it is still important to be discreet about your consumption at work. Opt for discreet consumption methods like vaporizers or edibles to minimize any potential stigma or distractions.

5. Communicate openly: If using cannabis at work is allowed in your workplace or industry, communicate openly with your colleagues and superiors about your cannabis use. This can help to foster a supportive and understanding work environment.

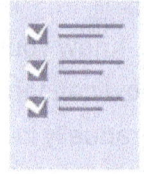

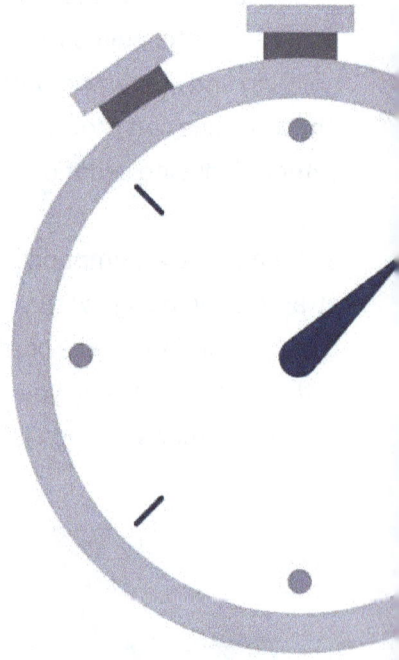

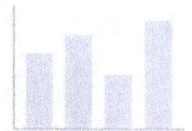

6. Take care of your wellness: Cannabis can be a valuable tool for enhancing wellness, but it is essential to prioritize self-care. Stay hydrated, eat nutritious meals, exercise regularly, and get enough sleep to ensure you are in the best possible state to excel in your professional endeavors.

Remember, using cannabis at work is a personal choice, and it may
not be suitable for everyone. It is important to consult with a
medical professional or cannabis expert to determine if it aligns
with your individual needs and circumstances.

By following these tips, professional men and women aged 30-75
can explore the potential benefits of cannabis while maintaining
productivity and wellness in their work lives. With responsible
consumption and a thoughtful approach, cannabis can become a
valuable tool for boosting productivity and enhancing overall well-
being in the modern professional world.

Balancing Cannabis Use with Other Wellness Practices

In today's fast-paced world, it can be challenging to find the right
balance between work, personal life, and overall well-being. As
professionals, we often strive for productivity and success, but it's
equally important to prioritize our mental and physical health.
Cannabis can play a role in enhancing our wellness, but it's
essential to strike a balance and incorporate it into a holistic
approach to self-care.

This subchapter explores how professional men and women, aged 30 to 75, can integrate cannabis use into their wellness practices effectively. By understanding the benefits of various cannabis strains and incorporating them alongside other wellness activities, we can optimize productivity and overall well-being.

To begin, it's crucial to acknowledge that cannabis is not a one-size-fits-all solution. Different strains have different effects, and selecting the right one for your needs is essential. This guidebook aims to provide professional individuals with the knowledge to make informed decisions about cannabis strains that can enhance their productivity and wellness.

Balancing cannabis use with other wellness practices involves finding synergy between various activities that promote well-being. For example, incorporating mindfulness and meditation techniques alongside cannabis use can help reduce stress and improve focus. Additionally, regular exercise and a healthy diet can complement the effects of cannabis, promoting a more balanced and energized state of being.

Furthermore, it's crucial to establish boundaries and set limits when it comes to cannabis use. Understanding the right dosage and scheduling usage can prevent potential negative impacts on productivity and overall well-being. Striving for moderation and self-awareness allows individuals to harness the benefits of cannabis while maintaining control over their professional and personal lives.

Ultimately, the goal of balancing cannabis use with other wellness practices is to achieve optimal productivity and well-being. By integrating cannabis into a comprehensive wellness routine that includes mindfulness, exercise, and a healthy lifestyle, professional men and women can unlock the full potential of their productivity while maintaining a healthy work-life balance.

In conclusion, this subchapter serves as a guide to help professional men and women navigate the world of cannabis while prioritizing their overall wellness. By understanding the benefits of different strains and integrating cannabis into a holistic approach to self-care, individuals can enhance their productivity and well-being. It's crucial to strike a balance, set boundaries, and incorporate other wellness practices to achieve optimal results. With the right knowledge and approach, cannabis can be a valuable tool for the modern professional looking to boost productivity and wellness.

Leveraging Cannabis for Long-Term Career Growth

In today's fast-paced and demanding professional world, finding ways to boost productivity and maintain overall wellness is crucial for long-term career growth. Surprisingly, cannabis can play an essential role in achieving these goals. With its diverse strains and therapeutic properties, this plant has the potential to revolutionize the modern professional's approach to productivity and well-being.

While many may associate cannabis solely with recreational use, it is important to recognize the medicinal benefits it offers. This subchapter aims to provide professional men and women, aged 30-75, with a comprehensive guide on leveraging cannabis strains to enhance their career growth.

Understanding the unique properties of various cannabis strains is essential for professionals seeking to maximize their productivity. Different strains have distinct effects on the mind and body, allowing individuals to strategically tailor their cannabis use to meet their specific needs. For instance, sativa strains are known for their energizing and uplifting effects, making them ideal for boosting focus and creativity during brainstorming sessions or overcoming mental blocks. On the other hand, indica strains provide relaxation and can be beneficial for stress relief after a long and demanding workday.

By carefully selecting the right strain and incorporating it into their daily routine, professionals can optimize their productivity and overall well-being. However, it is crucial to approach cannabis use responsibly and in moderation. Striking a balance between leveraging its benefits and maintaining a professional image is key.

This subchapter will also delve into the ways cannabis can enhance wellness and promote work-life balance. Stress and burnout are prevalent issues in the professional world, and cannabis can be a valuable tool in managing these challenges. Certain strains possess calming properties that can alleviate anxiety and promote a sense of relaxation, allowing professionals to recharge and maintain their mental and emotional well-being.

Furthermore, this guide will explore the potential of cannabis in enhancing creativity, problem-solving skills, and overall cognitive function. Research suggests that specific strains can stimulate the imagination and enhance divergent thinking, leading to innovative solutions and increased resourcefulness.

In conclusion, leveraging cannabis for long-term career growth is an untapped potential that professional men and women should explore. This subchapter aims to provide a comprehensive guide to help professionals navigate the vast world of cannabis strains, enabling them to boost productivity, enhance wellness, and achieve long-term success in their careers. By understanding the unique properties of each strain and using it responsibly, professionals can harness the power of cannabis to reach new heights in their professional lives.

06

Chapter 6: Legal and Ethical Considerations for Professionals

Understanding Cannabis Laws and Regulations

In recent years, there has been a surge of interest in cannabis as a means to enhance productivity and overall wellness. With the legalization of cannabis in many parts of the world, it is crucial for professional men and women aged 30-75 to have a clear understanding of the laws and regulations surrounding its use. This subchapter aims to provide a comprehensive overview of the legal landscape surrounding cannabis, ensuring that you can navigate this emerging industry with confidence.

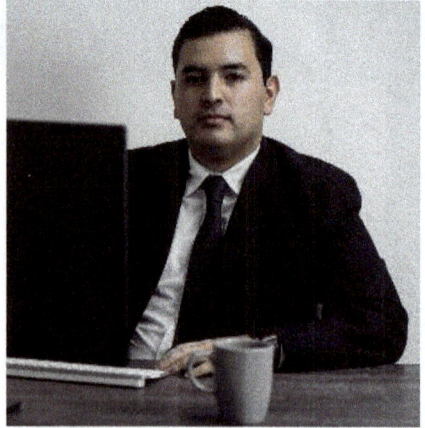

The first step towards understanding cannabis laws and regulations is to familiarize oneself with the legal status of cannabis in your region. Laws regarding cannabis can vary greatly from one jurisdiction to another, ranging from complete prohibition to full legalization. It is important to be aware of the specific regulations governing the possession, cultivation, and distribution of cannabis in your area, as well as any restrictions on its use in the workplace.

Cannabis Strains for the Modern Professional: A Guide to Boosting Productivity and Wellness

Furthermore, it is crucial to understand the different types of cannabis products available and how they are regulated. From dried flowers to edibles and concentrates, each product category may have its own set of rules governing production, labeling, and packaging.

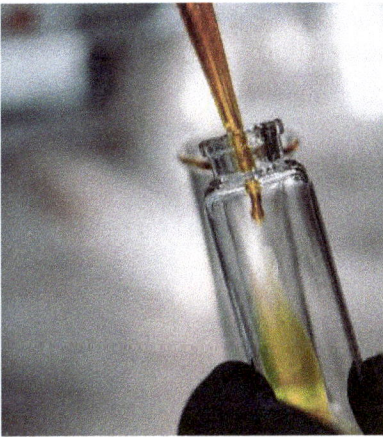

This knowledge will not only ensure compliance with the law but also enable you to make informed decisions when choosing cannabis products for your personal use.

In addition to legal considerations, it is essential to be aware of the potential health and safety risks associated with cannabis use. Understanding the potential side effects and interactions with other medications or substances is vital, especially for professionals who need to maintain optimal cognitive function and performance.

Familiarizing oneself with the recommended dosage, consumption methods, and potential risks will help mitigate any negative effects and ensure a safe and responsible cannabis experience.

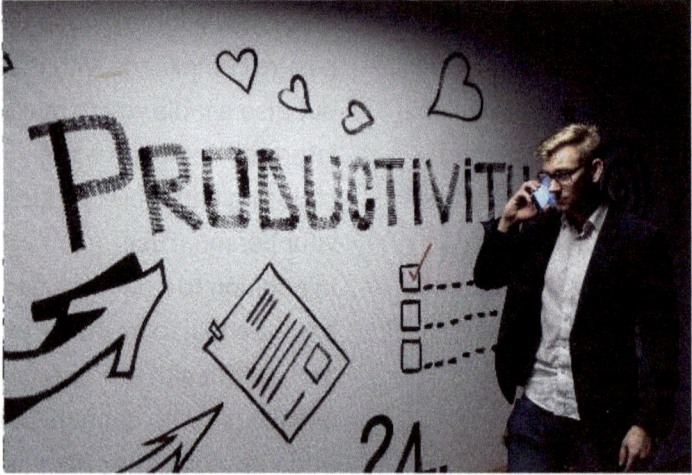

Lastly, staying informed about changes in cannabis laws and regulations is crucial in this rapidly evolving industry. As more research is conducted and societal attitudes shift, laws surrounding cannabis are subject to change. Regularly checking for updates and staying engaged with the latest news and developments will ensure that you are always up-to-date and can adapt your cannabis use accordingly.

By understanding the laws and regulations surrounding cannabis, professional men and women aged 30-75 can confidently incorporate cannabis into their lives while remaining compliant, safe, and responsible. This knowledge will empower you to make informed decisions about using cannabis to boost productivity and wellness, ensuring a positive and rewarding experience in this exciting new era of cannabis legalization.

Navigating Drug Testing and Employment Policies

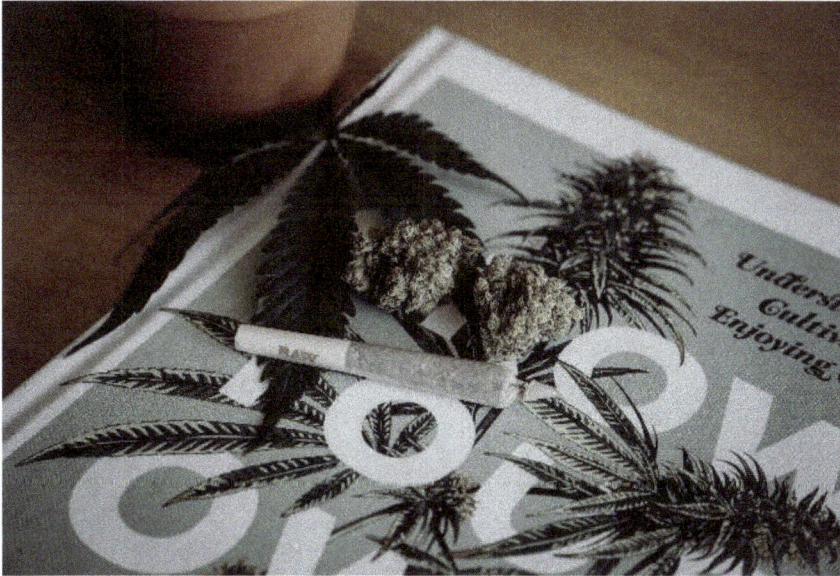

Cannabis Strains for the Modern Professional: A Guide to Boosting Productivity and Wellness

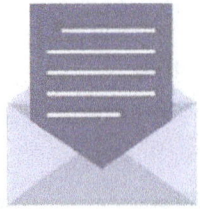

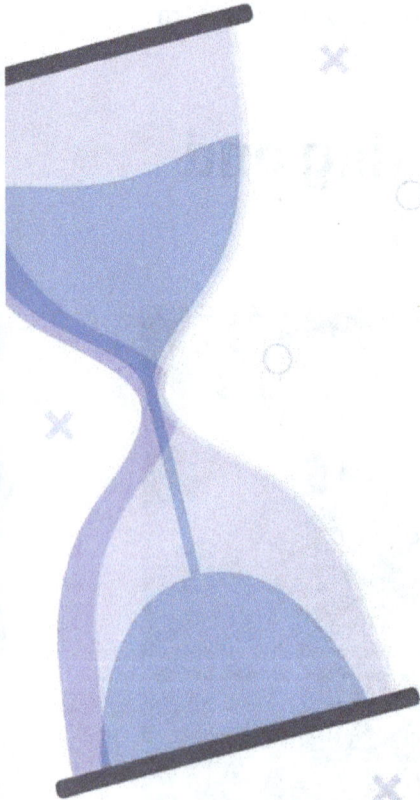

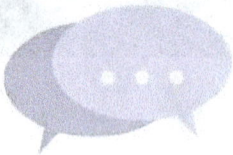

Drug testing and employment policies are important considerations for professionals, especially those who are interested in incorporating cannabis strains into their productivity and wellness routines. While cannabis has gained significant recognition for its potential health benefits, including stress reduction, pain management, and improved sleep, it is crucial to understand the implications of drug testing and company policies before incorporating cannabis into your daily life.

Drug testing is a common practice in many workplaces, and employers may have strict policies regarding the use of drugs, including cannabis. It is essential to familiarize yourself with your company's drug testing policy to ensure that you are aware of any potential consequences of using cannabis strains.

For professional men and women between the ages of 30 and 75, who are seeking to enhance their productivity and wellness, it is advisable to take a proactive approach in navigating drug testing and employment policies. Here are a few key points to consider:

1. Familiarize yourself with company policies: Take the time to read and understand your company's drug testing policy. Look for any specific guidelines or restrictions regarding cannabis use, including both recreational and medicinal purposes.

2. Communicate with your employer: If you are considering incorporating cannabis strains into your routine, it can be helpful to have an open and honest conversation with your employer. Discuss your intentions, the potential benefits you hope to achieve, and any concerns you may have about drug testing policies.

3. Explore alternative options: If your company has strict drug testing policies, it may be necessary to explore alternative wellness practices that can complement your goals without conflicting with employment policies. This could include mindfulness exercises, yoga, or other stress reduction techniques.

4. Stay informed about legal developments: Laws surrounding cannabis use are continually evolving. Stay up-to-date with the latest legal developments in your region to understand how they may impact your workplace drug testing policies.

Remember, while cannabis strains can offer many potential benefits for productivity and wellness, it is essential to be mindful of your workplace policies and regulations. By taking a proactive approach and staying informed, you can navigate drug testing and employment policies while still benefiting from the positive effects of cannabis strains on your overall well-being.

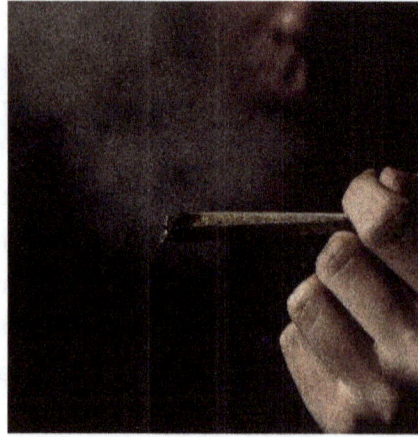

Addressing Stigma and Perception in Professional Environments

In recent years, the perception of cannabis has undergone a significant transformation. Once associated solely with recreational use and counterculture, cannabis has now emerged as a powerful tool for boosting productivity and wellness in professional environments. However, despite the growing acceptance of cannabis, stigma and negative perceptions still linger, particularly in professional settings.

This subchapter aims to address these concerns and provide guidance for professional men and women aged 30-75 who are interested in exploring the benefits of cannabis strains for their productivity and overall well-being.

First and foremost, it is essential to acknowledge the existing stigma surrounding cannabis. Many professionals worry that openly discussing their use of cannabis may compromise their reputation or career prospects. However, it is important to remember that perceptions are shifting rapidly. As more research emerges, highlighting the potential benefits of cannabis, professionals are beginning to recognize the value it can bring to their lives.

To navigate professional environments successfully, it is crucial to be well-informed about the different strains of cannabis available and their specific effects. Our Cannabis Strains for the Modern Professional guidebook serves as an invaluable resource in this regard. It provides comprehensive information on various strains, including their THC and CBD levels, terpene profiles, and potential benefits. Armed with this knowledge, professionals can make informed decisions about which strains are best suited to their individual needs, ensuring they experience the desired effects while maintaining their productivity and focus.

Furthermore, it is essential to adopt an open and transparent approach when discussing cannabis use with colleagues and superiors. By openly sharing the reasons behind their choice to incorporate cannabis into their routine, professionals can help dispel misconceptions and educate others about its potential benefits. This can foster a more accepting and understanding environment, ultimately reducing the stigma associated with cannabis use.

Lastly, it is crucial to emphasize responsible consumption. Professionals must prioritize moderation and self-regulation to ensure that cannabis enhances their productivity rather than hinders it. This involves understanding the appropriate dosage, setting clear boundaries, and being mindful of the specific effects different strains may have on their focus and attention.

In conclusion, addressing stigma and perception in professional environments is a crucial step towards unlocking the full potential of cannabis for productivity and wellness. By arming themselves with knowledge, adopting an open approach, and practicing responsible consumption, professional men and women aged 30-75 can confidently incorporate cannabis into their lives while maintaining their professionalism and achieving their goals.

Ethical Responsibilities and Considerations for Cannabis Use

As the popularity of cannabis continues to rise, it is crucial for professional men and women aged 30-75 to understand the ethical responsibilities and considerations that come with its use. While cannabis can provide numerous benefits for productivity and wellness, it is essential to approach its usage in a responsible and ethical manner.

First and foremost, it is crucial to recognize the legalities surrounding cannabis use in your jurisdiction. Laws regarding cannabis can vary significantly from one region to another, and it is vital to familiarize yourself with the regulations in your area. Ensuring that you are using cannabis within the confines of the law is not only ethically responsible but also crucial for avoiding any legal complications.

Another important ethical consideration is the impact of cannabis on your professional life. While cannabis can enhance productivity and overall well-being, it is crucial to assess how it may affect your work performance and relationships. It is essential to be mindful of the potential impairments that can arise from cannabis use and to ensure that it does not interfere with your ability to meet professional obligations or negatively impact your interactions with colleagues or clients.

Open and honest communication is also a key ethical responsibility when it comes to cannabis use. If you choose to incorporate cannabis into your wellness routine, it is crucial to have transparent conversations with those who may be affected, such as your family, close friends, or employers. By openly discussing your cannabis use, you provide an opportunity for understanding, support, and potentially even education for those who may have misconceptions about its benefits and effects.

Additionally, ethical cannabis use involves considering the sustainability and ethical practices of the industry. As a responsible consumer, it is vital to support businesses that prioritize sustainable cultivation methods, fair trade practices, and environmentally friendly packaging. By making conscious choices about where you source your cannabis products, you contribute to the overall ethical development of the industry.

In conclusion, as professional men and women seeking to enhance productivity and wellness through cannabis use, it is essential to recognize the ethical responsibilities and considerations that come with it. By adhering to legalities, assessing its impact on your professional life, engaging in open communication, and supporting ethical practices within the industry, you can ensure that your cannabis use aligns with your values and contributes positively to your overall well-being.

07

Chapter 7: Resources and Recommendations For Cannabis Strain Selection

Trusted Sources for Strain Information

When it comes to navigating the vast world of cannabis strains, it's crucial to have access to reliable and trustworthy sources for strain information. As a professional seeking to incorporate cannabis into your life to enhance productivity and wellness, having accurate and up-to-date knowledge about different strains is essential.

This subchapter explores some of the most trusted sources for strain information, ensuring that you can make informed decisions about which strains will best suit your specific needs.

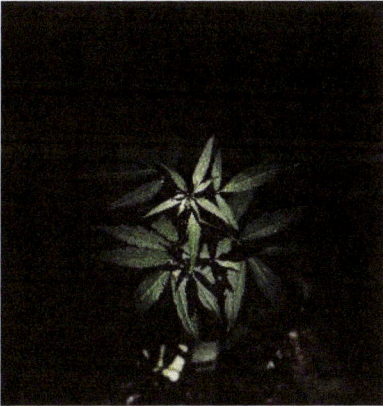

Cannabis Strains for the Modern Professional: A Guide to Boosting Productivity and Wellness

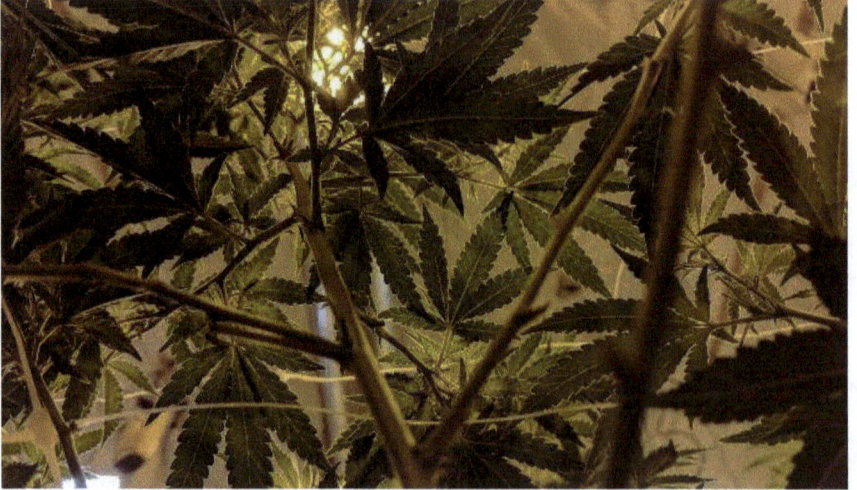

1. Cannabis Dispensaries: Local dispensaries are often an excellent place to start your search for strain information. Knowledgeable budtenders can provide valuable insights into various strains and their effects. They can guide you through the different options available and help you find strains that align with your professional goals and lifestyle.

2. Online Strain Databases: Numerous online platforms specialize in providing comprehensive strain information. Websites like Leafly, Weedmaps, and AllBud offer extensive strain databases that include detailed descriptions, user reviews, and even information about the strains' origins and genetics. These platforms also allow users to search for strains based on specific effects, flavors, and medicinal properties, making it easier to find strains tailored to your preferences.

3. Cannabis Magazines and Publications: Many reputable magazines and publications focus on cannabis strain reviews and provide in-depth analysis of different strains. Publications such as High Times, Cannabis Now, and Marijuana Business Magazine often feature articles written by experts in the field, discussing the unique characteristics and effects of various strains. These sources can be a valuable resource for expanding your strain knowledge.

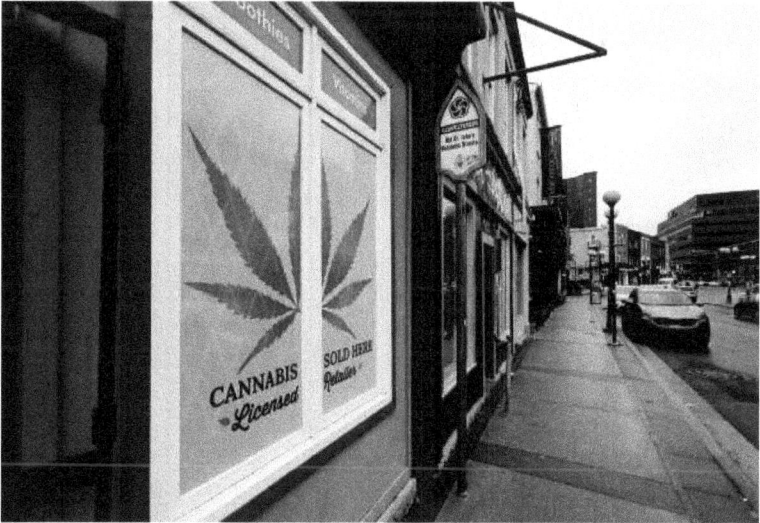

4. Cannabis Conferences and Events: Attending cannabis conferences and events is an excellent opportunity to learn about new strains and gain insights from industry professionals. These gatherings often feature panel discussions, workshops, and presentations by experts who share their expertise on strains and their applications.

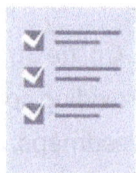

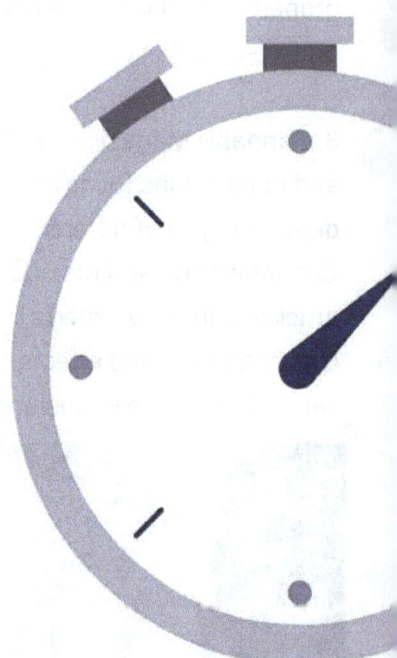

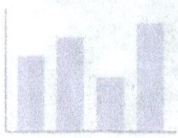

By participating in these events, you can stay up-to-date with the latest developments in the cannabis industry and discover new strains that may enhance your professional life.

Remember, it's crucial to cross-reference information from different sources to ensure accuracy and reliability. The cannabis landscape is constantly evolving, with new strains being introduced regularly. By utilizing trusted sources for strain information, you can make informed decisions and find the strains that best align with your goals of boosting productivity and overall wellness in your professional life.

Online Tools and Apps for Cannabis Strain Selection

In today's digital age, technology has transformed the way we navigate the world, and cannabis is no exception. Gone are the days when selecting a cannabis strain was a daunting task solely reliant on word-of-mouth recommendations or trial and error. Thanks to the emergence of online tools and apps, cannabis strain selection has become more accessible, efficient, and tailored to individual preferences.

For professional men and women aged 30-75, who are seeking to enhance their productivity and overall wellness with cannabis, these online tools and apps can be invaluable resources. Whether you are a seasoned cannabis enthusiast or a newcomer to the world of cannabis, these tools will help you make informed decisions when choosing the right strain for your specific needs.

Cannabis Strains for the Modern Professional: A Guide to Boosting Productivity and Wellness

One of the most popular online tools is the cannabis strain database. These databases compile comprehensive information about various strains, including their effects, flavors, THC and CBD levels, and medical benefits. With just a few clicks, you can access a wealth of knowledge and gain a deeper understanding of each strain's properties. This allows you to narrow down your options based on your desired effects, such as increased focus, relaxation, or pain relief.

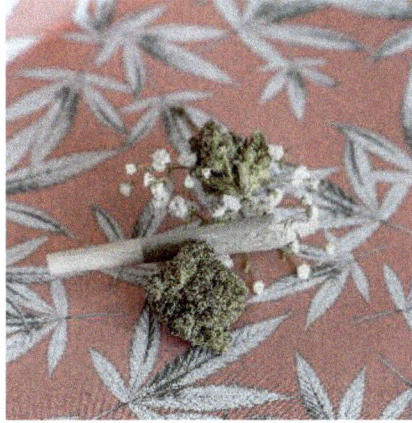

Moreover, there are mobile apps specifically designed to assist in strain selection. These apps often feature user-friendly interfaces, strain reviews, and personalized recommendations based on your preferences and previous experiences.

They may also provide dosage guidelines, strain comparisons, and even track your cannabis consumption history.

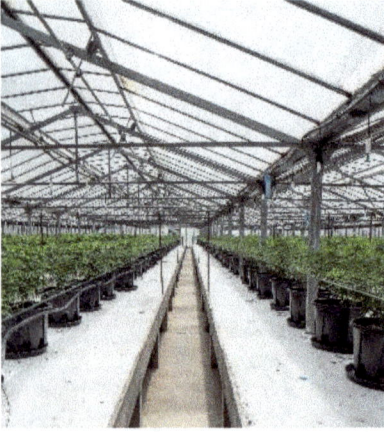

In addition to strain databases and mobile apps, online communities and forums dedicated to cannabis enthusiasts offer a wealth of information and advice. These platforms allow you to connect with like-minded individuals, share experiences, and seek recommendations.

Engaging in these communities can provide valuable insights and recommendations from experienced users, helping you broaden your knowledge and discover new strains that align with your goals.

As a professional seeking to optimize your productivity and wellness, leveraging online tools and apps for cannabis strain selection is an excellent way to elevate your cannabis experience. With the knowledge and convenience offered by these resources, you can confidently navigate the vast world of cannabis strains, ensuring that you find the perfect match for your needs and preferences.

Remember, the key to responsible cannabis use is informed decision-making. By utilizing these online tools and apps, you can make well-informed choices, leading to a more productive, balanced, and fulfilling lifestyle.

Recommendations for Specific Professional Situations and Needs

In this subchapter, we will explore specific professional situations and needs that can benefit from the use of cannabis strains. As professional men and women aged 30-75, you understand the importance of finding ways to boost productivity and wellness in your work and personal lives. Cannabis strains offer a unique solution that can help you achieve these goals, provided they are used responsibly and legally.

1. Stress and Anxiety Relief: High-stress jobs can take a toll on your mental well-being. Consider trying strains known for their calming effects, such as Blue Dream or Granddaddy Purple. These strains can help alleviate stress and anxiety, allowing you to focus better and feel more relaxed throughout the day.

2. Focus and Concentration: Some professionals may struggle with maintaining focus and concentration, especially during long hours of work. Look for strains like Green Crack or Durban Poison, known for their energizing and uplifting effects. These strains can provide a boost of mental clarity and focus, helping you stay on task and be more productive.

3. Creative Thinking: For those in creative fields or professions that require innovative thinking, certain cannabis strains can enhance your creativity. Strains like Sour Diesel or Jack Herer are known for their stimulating effects, allowing your mind to wander and explore new ideas.

4. Pain and Inflammation Management: Many professionals may suffer from chronic pain or inflammation due to their work environment or long hours spent sitting. Consider strains like ACDC or Harlequin, which have high CBD content and are known for their pain-relieving properties. These strains can help manage pain and reduce inflammation, allowing you to focus on your work with minimal discomfort.

5. Sleep Aid: Quality sleep is crucial for professionals to perform at their best. If you struggle with insomnia or have trouble winding down after a long day, strains like Northern Lights or Purple Kush can promote relaxation and aid in achieving a restful night's sleep. Remember, it is essential to consult with a healthcare professional or a knowledgeable budtender to find the right strain and dosage for your specific needs. Additionally, always ensure that you are using cannabis responsibly and legally in your jurisdiction.

By exploring these recommendations for specific professional situations and needs, you can harness the potential of cannabis strains to boost your productivity and overall wellness.

Building a Personalized Cannabis Strain Collection

In this subchapter, we will explore the art of building a personalized cannabis strain collection, specifically tailored for professional men and women in the age range of 30-75. As the cannabis industry continues to evolve and gain acceptance, it is crucial to understand the different strains available and how to curate a collection that enhances productivity and wellness.

1. Understanding Cannabis Strains:
To begin, it is essential to grasp the fundamental differences
between various cannabis strains. CBD-dominant strains offer
therapeutic benefits without the psychoactive effects, making
them ideal for daytime use. THC-dominant strains, on the other
hand, provide a more euphoric experience, perfect for relaxation
after a long day. By understanding the unique properties and
effects of each strain, you can create a balanced collection that
caters to your specific needs.

2. Identifying Personal Goals:
Before embarking on building your cannabis strain collection, it is
crucial to identify your personal goals. Are you seeking stress relief,
pain management, or increased focus? By pinpointing your desired
outcomes, you can select strains that align with your intentions.
This personalized approach ensures that your cannabis collection
becomes a valuable tool for enhancing productivity and wellness.

3. Research and Experimentation:
Building a cannabis strain collection is an ongoing process that
requires research and experimentation. Familiarize yourself with
reputable sources to learn about the different strains available,
their effects, and potential benefits. Experiment with various
strains to determine which ones resonate with you the most. Keep
a journal to document your experiences and track the effects of
each strain. This will help you refine your collection over time and
make informed decisions about which strains to include.

4. Diversifying Your Collection:
To create a well-rounded cannabis strain collection, it is essential to diversify. Consider including a range of strains with different THC and CBD ratios to cater to various needs and preferences. Additionally, explore strains with terpene profiles that align with your desired effects. Terpenes, the aromatic compounds found in cannabis, play a significant role in the overall experience and can further enhance the therapeutic benefits.

5. Responsible Consumption:
Lastly, it is crucial to approach cannabis consumption responsibly. Start with low doses, especially when trying new strains, to gauge their effects on your mind and body. Observe how each strain interacts with your unique biology and adjust your consumption accordingly. Remember, moderation is key to harnessing the productivity and wellness benefits of cannabis without impairing your professional life.

Building a personalized cannabis strain collection is an exciting journey that allows professional men and women to optimize their productivity and wellness. By understanding the different strains, identifying personal goals, conducting thorough research, experimenting, and consuming responsibly, you can curate a collection that enhances your professional and personal life.

08

Conclusion: Embracing Cannabis as a Tool for Professional Success and Wellness

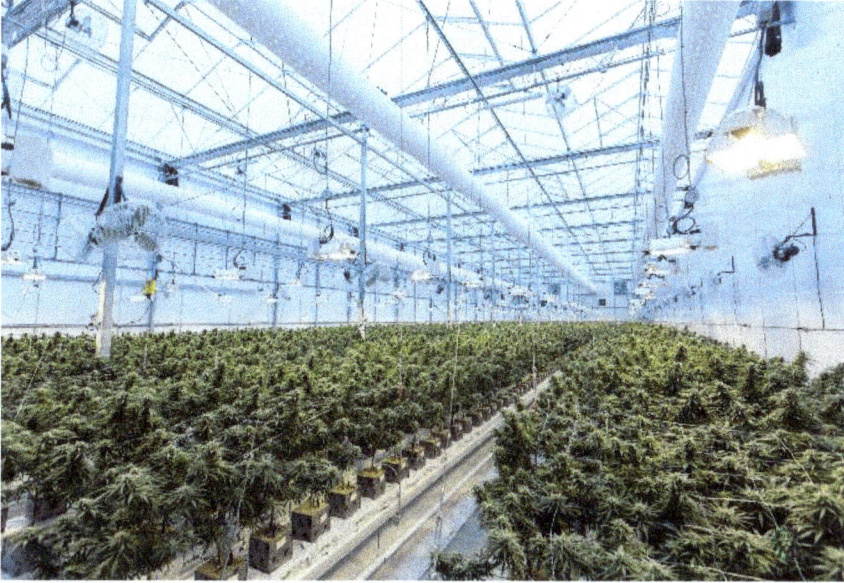

Summarizing Key Points and Takeaways

In this subchapter, we will summarize the key points and takeaways from the book "Cannabis Strains for the Modern Professional: A Guide to Boosting Productivity and Wellness." Whether you are a professional man or woman between the ages of 30 and 75, this cannabis strain guide book is tailored to help you navigate the world of cannabis and enhance your productivity and wellness.

Cannabis Strains for the Modern Professional: A Guide to Boosting Productivity and Wellness

First and foremost, it is essential to understand that cannabis can be a powerful tool when used responsibly and appropriately. The book emphasizes the importance of finding the right strain that suits your specific needs and goals. Each strain has its unique characteristics, such as THC and CBD content, terpene profiles, and effects. By understanding these elements, you can choose the perfect strain that aligns with your desired outcomes.

Furthermore, the book highlights the significance of using cannabis as a means to boost productivity rather than hinder it. It explores various strains specifically curated for professional individuals, taking into account their energy-boosting, focus-enhancing, and stress-relieving properties. The goal is to optimize your performance while maintaining a balanced and healthy lifestyle.

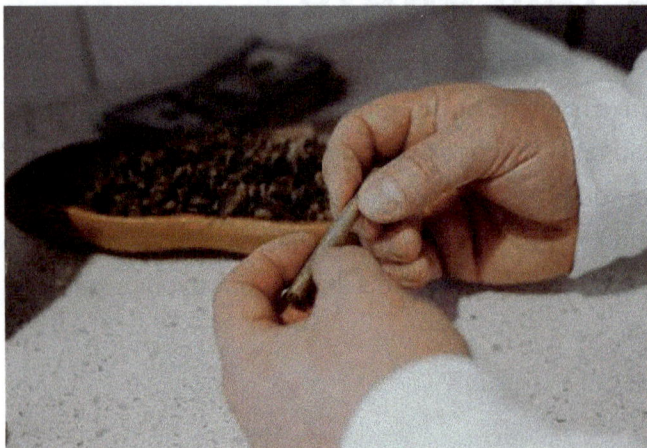

Cannabis Strains for the Modern Professional: A Guide to Boosting Productivity and Wellness

Additionally, the book addresses the importance of responsible consumption and dosage control. It provides guidelines and recommendations on how to start with lower doses and gradually increase as needed. It advises against overconsumption, which can lead to diminished productivity and unwanted side effects.

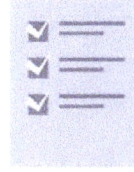

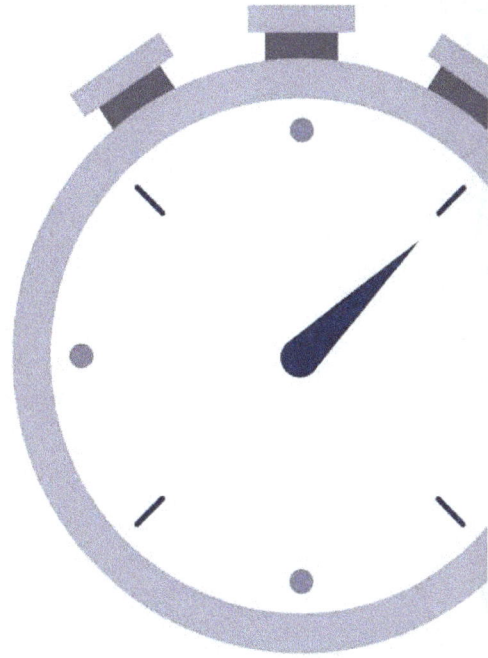

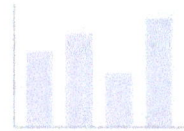

Cannabis Strains for the Modern Professional: A Guide to Boosting Productivity and Wellness

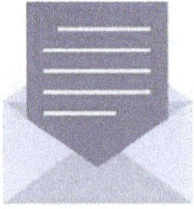

Moreover, this guide book takes a holistic approach by discussing the potential wellness benefits of cannabis. It explores strains that may alleviate symptoms of anxiety, depression, chronic pain, and other common ailments experienced by professionals. By incorporating cannabis into your wellness routine, you can potentially enhance your overall well-being and quality of life.

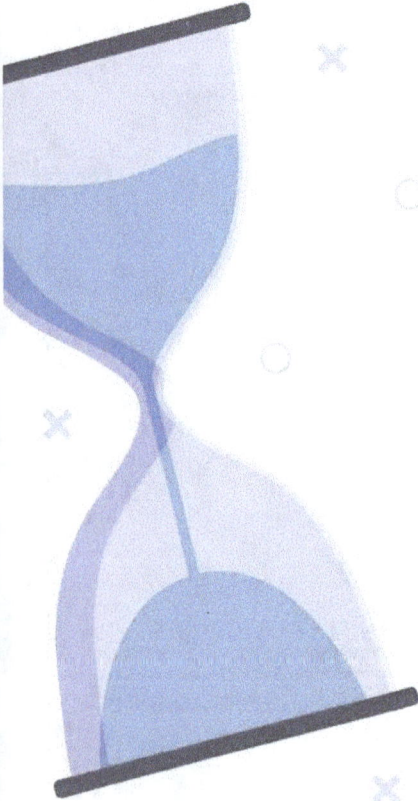

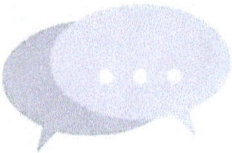

Lastly, the book acknowledges the importance of staying informed about laws and regulations surrounding cannabis use. It provides insights into the legal landscape, ensuring that readers can make informed decisions that comply with their local jurisdiction.
In conclusion, "Cannabis Strains for the Modern Professional: A Guide to Boosting Productivity and Wellness" is a comprehensive resource tailored to professional men and women aged 30-75 seeking to explore the world of cannabis. By summarizing the key points and takeaways, this subchapter ensures that you have a clear understanding of how to choose the right strains, use cannabis responsibly, optimize productivity, and enhance your overall wellness.

Encouraging Responsible Cannabis Use

In the rapidly evolving landscape of cannabis legalization, it is crucial to approach the topic of consumption with responsibility and mindfulness. This subchapter aims to guide professional men and women, aged 30-75, on the path of responsible cannabis use, ensuring productivity and wellness are at the forefront of their experience.

Cannabis Strains for the Modern Professional: A Guide to Boosting Productivity and Wellness

1. Understanding Moderation: While cannabis can provide numerous benefits, it is essential to recognize the importance of moderation. This means finding a balance between enjoying the benefits of cannabis and maintaining a productive and fulfilling life. By understanding the appropriate dosage, frequency, and timing of consumption, professionals can integrate cannabis into their lives without compromising their responsibilities.

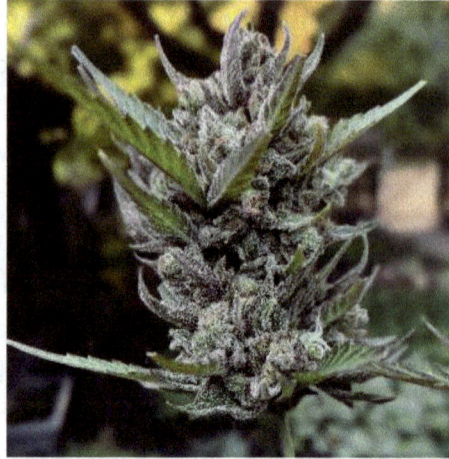

2. Identifying Strains for Productivity:
One of the key aspects of responsible cannabis use is selecting strains that enhance productivity rather than hinder it. This chapter will introduce readers to a variety of cannabis strains that promote focus, creativity, and energy. By understanding the unique effects of different strains, professionals can make informed decisions and choose strains that align with their specific needs and goals.

3. Mindful Consumption Techniques:
Exploring mindful consumption techniques can significantly contribute to responsible cannabis use. This subchapter will delve into methods such as microdosing, which involves taking small amounts of cannabis to experience subtle effects without impairment.
Additionally, we will explore alternative consumption methods such as vaporizers, edibles, and topical applications, each offering different benefits and effects.

4. Creating a Safe and Comfortable Environment:
To foster responsible cannabis use, it is essential to create a safe and comfortable environment for consumption. This includes identifying suitable locations, ensuring privacy, and understanding legal regulations in your area. Furthermore, we will discuss the importance of open communication with loved ones and colleagues to alleviate any potential concerns and encourage a supportive atmosphere.

5. Personal Wellness and Self-Care:
Lastly, responsible cannabis use goes hand in hand with personal wellness and self-care. This chapter will emphasize the importance of maintaining a holistic approach to well-being, which includes physical exercise, a balanced diet, and quality sleep. By integrating these practices alongside cannabis use, professionals can optimize their productivity and overall sense of wellness.

In conclusion, the subchapter on "Encouraging Responsible Cannabis Use" within the book "Cannabis Strains for the Modern Professional: A Guide to Boosting Productivity and Wellness" aims to provide professional men and women aged 30-75 with the knowledge and tools necessary for responsible cannabis consumption. By understanding moderation, selecting appropriate strains, practicing mindful consumption techniques, creating a safe environment, and prioritizing personal wellness, individuals can navigate the world of cannabis with confidence, enhancing their productivity and overall well-being.

Inspiring Professional Men and Women to Harness the Benefits of Cannabis for Productivity and Wellness.

In today's fast-paced and demanding professional world, it's no surprise that many individuals are seeking ways to enhance their productivity and overall wellness. While cannabis may not be the first solution that comes to mind, it is increasingly being recognized for its potential to improve focus, creativity, and overall well-being. This subchapter aims to empower professional men and women, aged 30-75, with the knowledge and guidance needed to harness the benefits of cannabis strains for their productivity and wellness.

As a professional, you understand the importance of maintaining a high level of productivity without compromising your well-being. Cannabis strains have evolved significantly over the years, providing a wide variety of options tailored to your specific needs.

This guidebook will help you navigate the world of cannabis strains, offering insights into their different effects, dosages, and consumption methods. By understanding the science behind cannabis and its interaction with your body, you can make informed decisions that align with your professional goals.

One of the key benefits of cannabis lies in its ability to enhance focus and creativity. Whether you're a writer, artist, or entrepreneur, certain strains can unlock your creative potential, allowing you to think outside the box and approach challenges with a fresh perspective. By incorporating cannabis into your daily routine, you can tap into a new level of productivity that was previously untapped.

In addition to productivity, wellness is a crucial aspect of professional success. Cannabis strains can be a powerful tool in managing stress, anxiety, and even physical ailments. From relieving work-related stress to alleviating chronic pain, there is a strain tailored to address your specific wellness needs. By prioritizing your well-being, you can ensure longevity and sustained success in your professional journey.

This subchapter will delve into the different cannabis strains that are ideal for professionals, exploring their unique properties and potential applications. It will provide guidance on dosage, consumption methods, and how to incorporate cannabis into your daily routine effectively. Through the knowledge shared in this guidebook, you will be equipped to make informed decisions that optimize your productivity and well-being.

As a professional, it's essential to stay ahead of the curve and explore innovative approaches to enhance your productivity and overall wellness. Cannabis strains offer a natural and holistic solution that can revolutionize the way you work and live. Embrace the potential of cannabis and unlock the doors to a more productive and fulfilling professional life.

09

Looking Ahead

The Future of Cannabis As we approach the end of our comprehensive journey through the world of cannabis, it's clear that this is not the conclusion but rather a new beginning. The cannabis industry is evolving at an unprecedented pace, with scientific discoveries, legal reforms, and cultural shifts shaping its future. This final section explores emerging trends, potential challenges, and exciting opportunities in the cannabis landscape, offering a glimpse into what might lie ahead and setting the stage for a deeper exploration in a potential second book. The Next Frontier in Cannabis Research Scientific research into cannabis is burgeoning, shedding light on its myriad therapeutic potentials beyond what we've already discovered. The exploration of minor cannabinoids, such as cannabigerol (CBG) and cannabinol (CBN), is gaining momentum, promising new treatments for conditions ranging from neurodegenerative diseases to insomnia.

Furthermore, the advancement in genetic engineering and
cultivation techniques is poised to produce strains with tailored
cannabinoid profiles, maximizing therapeutic benefits while
minimizing adverse effects. This burgeoning field of study not only
expands our understanding of cannabis but also opens the door to
personalized medicine, where treatments could be customized to
individual genetic profiles and specific health conditions. Legal
Landscapes and Social Impacts Globally, the legal status of
cannabis is in flux, with numerous countries and states
reconsidering their stance on prohibition. This shifting legal
landscape presents both opportunities and challenges. On one
hand, legalization and decriminalization can lead to significant
economic benefits, reduced incarceration rates, and increased
scientific research.

On the other hand, these changes raise questions about regulation, quality control, and the social implications of increased accessibility. The next phase of legal reform will need to address these complex issues, balancing the economic and medicinal benefits of cannabis with concerns about public health and safety. The Cultural Shift Cannabis is experiencing a cultural renaissance, moving away from stigmatization and towards acceptance and normalization. This shift is reflected in mainstream media, lifestyle products, and even in the integration of cannabis into wellness routines. As cannabis becomes more ingrained in daily life, understanding its cultural significance and impact becomes increasingly important. The role of cannabis in art, music, and community building, as well as its influence on popular culture and social movements, will likely be key themes explored in future discussions and writings. Toward a Sustainable Future.

Sustainability in cannabis cultivation and production is becoming a pressing concern. As the industry grows, so does its environmental footprint. Future innovations will need to focus on eco-friendly practices, from reducing water and energy consumption to minimizing waste. The development of sustainable packaging solutions and the adoption of organic farming practices are just the beginning. The cannabis industry has the potential to lead by example, demonstrating how businesses can thrive while respecting and preserving the environment. The Global Cannabis Economy The international trade of cannabis and cannabis-derived products is set to expand, transforming the industry into a global powerhouse.

This evolution will require navigating complex international laws and regulations, but it also opens up a world of possibilities for cultural exchange, economic development, and global partnerships. Understanding the dynamics of the global cannabis market will be crucial for entrepreneurs, investors, and policymakers alike. As we look to the horizon, the potential for a second book becomes evident. There's so much more to explore, from the intricacies of global legalization efforts to the cutting-edge of cannabis science and the ongoing cultural revolution. The future of cannabis is bright, and it's a journey I look forward to continuing with you. Thank you for joining me on this exploration of cannabis. As we close this chapter, let's remain open-minded, curious, and compassionate, ready to embrace the opportunities and challenges that lie ahead. The conversation about cannabis is far from over; in many ways, it's just getting started.

This book is dedicated to the pioneers, the dreamers, the cultivators, and the advocates. To those who have paved the way for cannabis acceptance, fought for its legalization, and worked tirelessly to demystify its usage, we owe our deepest gratitude. Marlo Richardson, in partnership with Just Mary Cannabis Brands, extends this guide as a tribute to the enduring spirit of exploration and enlightenment within the cannabis community. Our journey is not merely about enjoying the myriad strains and their unique effects; it's about understanding, respect, and appreciation for the plant that brings us together. To our readers, whether you're taking your first step into the world of cannabis or you're a seasoned aficionado looking to deepen your knowledge, this guide is for you. May it inspire curiosity, encourage responsible exploration, and foster a greater appreciation for the art and science of cannabis cultivation and enjoyment. Let this book serve as a beacon for the ongoing journey towards understanding, acceptance, and love for cannabis. Here's to the endless pursuit of knowledge, the joy of discovery, and the unbreakable bond of a community united by a leaf.

Thank you to my family for allowing me the love and space to build and create.

Dr. Marlo Richardson and Just Mary Cannabis Brands

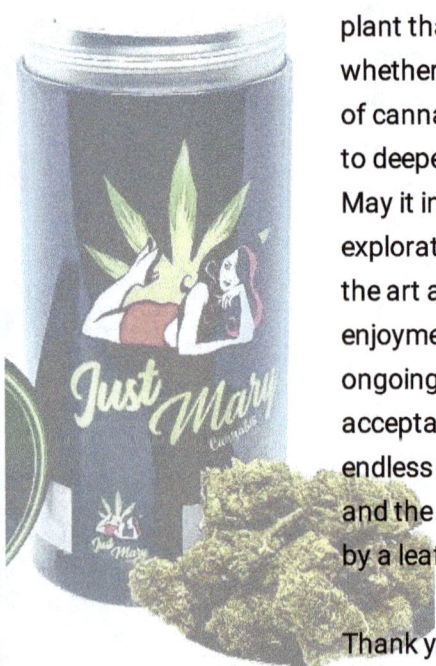

www.ingramcontent.com/pod-product-compliance
Lightning Source LLC
Chambersburg PA
CBHW070126030426
42335CB00016B/2278